JAMES J. O'CONNELL, M.D.

STORIES
FROM THE
SHADOWS

REFLECTIONS OF A STREET DOCTOR

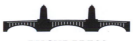

BHCHP PRESS

www.bhchp.org

Cover photo © Rick Friedman

Rick is a world-renowned photographer who accompanied Dr. O'Connell and Pine Street Inn van supervisor Leo Adorno on their night outreach duties. The photograph shows Dr. O'Connell and Leo having just stepped out of the van to examine an unconscious patient.

www.rickfriedman.com

Patient names and identifying details have been changed to protect the privacy of the individuals.

ISBN 978-0-692-41234-3

Library of Congress Control Number: 2015939222

Printed in the United States of America

Fourth Edition

To Gabriella

Contents

Foreword

You hold in your hands a precious gem. For this volume instantly and irrevocably transports you into a fascinating universe of individuals usually invisible to us. They are often faceless and nameless, lost in plain sight, and forced to live on the fringes of society. But this volume makes unforgettable those who are usually forgotten. The riveting stories presented here capture each life in such moving and vivid detail that you will be forever changed.

For too long, our society has been confounded in attempts to solve the challenge of homelessness. A tumultuous array of forces—poverty, illiteracy, mental illness, substance abuse, violence, and discrimination, among others—have conspired to create this challenge. In fact, such forces have left thousands of vulnerable people teetering on the fault lines of our society. The many issues involved have traditionally exasperated clinicians, defied policymakers, and often generated feelings of hopelessness for all involved.

But 30 years ago, the Boston Health Care for the Homeless Program (BHCHP) was born to bring hope to a situation so many considered hopeless. BHCHP heeded the words of the late Reverend William Sloane Coffin, who once said we should be "concerned most with those that society counted least and put last." In July 1985, a small group of seven professionals banded together to launch dedicated and coordinated clinical services for homeless people. They just wanted to serve. And by committing to the mission of BHCHP, they started a revolution.

The BHCHP founders insisted that their work be viewed as a commitment to social justice rather than as charity. They implemented a broad approach that bridged the worlds of medicine and public health, serving as the "glue" to link hospitals and health centers to shelters and homeless-service providers. They emphasized the coordination of primary care with mental health and substance-abuse services. And they built trust between the clinician and the client through extraordinary patience and perseverance.

Now, three decades later, BHCHP has grown to become the largest and most comprehensive freestanding Health Care for the Homeless program in the country. We can all marvel at a long list of pioneering accomplishments. For example, BHCHP became the first federally qualified health center made possible through funding from the Health Resources and Services Administration (HRSA) of the US Department of Health and Human Services (HHS). And by opening the Barbara McInnis House, BHCHP established the critical concept of medical respite care that prevents hospitalized patients from being discharged directly back to the streets.

In addition, in 1996 BHCHP created the first electronic medical system for homeless care that coordinates care and monitors quality measures across two hospitals and more than 65 shelter and street clinics. BHCHP has also promoted widespread insurance coverage for homeless persons as well as the provision of key preventive services (such as flu shots, certain cancer screenings, and care for homeless HIV-infected persons). It published the first ever *Manual of Communicable Diseases and Common Problems in Shelters and on the Streets* in 1994, followed by a second edition in 2005. And through it all, BHCHP has grown from 7 to 400 full-time employees and now serves over 12,000 homeless men, women, and children each year in Boston.

But despite the remarkable progress, this volume reminds us why the need for BHCHP remains overwhelming. In this book, we can feel that unmet need by peering into the world of Dr. Jim O'Connell. Jim has not only led BHCHP as president from the beginning but has also dedicated his life to those struggling for simple shelter and a warm meal. Over the decades, Jim felt compelled to capture many human vignettes of life on the streets through unforgettable snippets of writing. In fact, he has compiled dozens of these stories, with over 30 of them presented here. Some found their way into President's Reports to the BHCHP Board of Directors. Never intending to publish any of these, Jim initially filed many of them away in a shoebox. Fortunately for us, these stories have now been unearthed, drawing back the curtain on some extraordinary human tales.

In each story, the homeless lose their anonymity (although some only have a first name or a nickname). Nothing is routine in this world; nothing is orderly or reasoned. We meet people wrestling with demons, sometimes conversing with voices only they can hear. We agonize with a veteran who develops head and neck cancer soon after celebrating a year of sobriety. We marvel as Jim swaps thoughts on sophisticated theories with a homeless philosophy expert. And we are invited in as Jim trades literary insights with a homeless college professor.

Many are desperate. One man reminisces movingly about his beloved grandmother and aunt, only to be crushed to death by an SUV a short time later. Some die alone, with no one claiming their bodies for days or weeks on end.

And sometimes the stories occur within the backdrop of the march of American history. For example, one story takes place during the 1988 presidential election between George Bush and Michael Dukakis. Another takes place on September 11, 2001. Still another occurs soon after the 2013 Boston Marathon bombings. In each vignette, regardless of the national events of the moment, each person struggles to find some sense of meaning and stability amidst the jarring juxtapositions of their lives. Together, Jim and his colleagues have a personal and enduring relationship with them all.

I am so proud of BHCHP, and I am so proud of Jim. We first met several decades ago when we were both young physicians in training at Massachusetts General Hospital (MGH). At the time, Jim was fresh out of Harvard Medical School, just starting his internship—and I was only a few years ahead, a hematology-oncology fellow. Jim immediately made an impression upon me. His quiet brilliance was only matched by his utter modesty and humility. He also had that wonderful disarming smile, completely lacking the haughty façade of the stereotypical Ivy League physician. Jim's fundamental decency and genuine integrity came shining through every human encounter. It was clear Jim was a gift. He just wanted to serve.

We quickly bonded and became fast friends. In 1985, upon the completion of our MGH training, we met for a quick lunch in the spartan hospital cafeteria to share our plans for the future. When I asked Jim about next steps in his career, he humbly replied: "Well, they are establishing a new Health Care for the Homeless Program here in Boston and I think I will try to help." That was it. No long speeches. No ponderous pronouncements. Just a brief sentence, powerful in its simplicity. I remember being stunned by the enormity of his message. I couldn't even begin to fathom the overwhelming ramifications of such a challenge. Who could possibly know what the future would have in store?

In no time, Jim began to make his mark as one of the most extraordinary healers of our generation. Unlike the typical physician in a white coat waiting for daytime patients to arrive in the office, Jim and his new colleagues rode the van into the night, seeking to comfort those without a home. Those he cared for were eking out existences on a sidewalk, at a racetrack, under a bridge, or in a T station. Jim understood, of course, that the challenge was daunting. But he also knew that by being a "witness to human vulnerability," he could offer a soothing presence—one that affirmed each life as part of the great unfolding story that we all share, the meaning of which we can scarcely fathom.

At work, Jim is most comfortable dressed in blue jeans, and greets one and all with a hug and a warm smile. His contribution to patient care often starts with the offer of a hot bowl of soup or a soothing footbath to someone in need. Regularly, he will examine a fallen patient while crouching in the darkness on the street, literally on his knees, armed with only a dim flashlight. He often notes the bitter irony of vulnerable people dying in the shadows of Boston's most powerful institutions—on the grates of the Boston Public Library, propped up against the walls of MGH, or within steps of the city's many upscale hotels. He makes these observations without anger but rather with gentle passion and quiet compassion. Jim personifies both qualities: the root of the term "passion" means "to suffer" and "compassion" means "to suffer with."

And when I think of Jim and BHCHP, I often think of the words of theologian Father Henri Nouwen: "Compassion...asks us to go where it hurts, to enter into places of pain, to share in brokenness, fear, confusion and anguish...compassion means going directly to those people and places where suffering is most acute and building a home there... Compassion means full immersion in the condition of being human...(there is)...deep conviction that through compassion, our humanity grows into its fullness."

My friendship with Jim became even more precious during my time as Massachusetts Commissioner of Public Health. Then, I was privileged to see his inspiring work, up close and personally. I became reacquainted with the miracles of hope regularly delivered by him and BHCHP. I treasured the extraordinary care he and his wonderful colleagues provided at dozens of sites in metropolitan Boston. And whenever Jim would ask if there were ways he could help me in my job, I would reply that he was already doing enough by inspiring us all to be better healers. I was reminded time and again that Jim was a gift. I felt only gratitude that we were able to share our journey together.

One particularly harsh winter back then, about a dozen people froze to death on the streets of Boston. It was a shameful chapter of our state's public health history. As Commissioner I convened an emergency task force to generate a public health response. I am grateful for the dozens of committed professionals, from BHCHP and elsewhere, who joined in this venture.

Through a series of task-force meetings that extended over several years, I was honored to work through this crisis with the tremendous guidance and advice of Jim. In fact, I quickly came to realize that the meetings would proceed most smoothly if each one began with a report from him. Jim knew by name those who had perished, having personally cared for all of them. In his opening reports, he told stories of their personalities, their lives, their hopes, and their struggles. He brought the humanity back into the discussion. Jim always started us off on the right track and with the right tone. And as I watched Jim in action, I marveled that over the years he really hadn't changed at all. His passion and compassion and uncommon decency continued to shine for all to see.

As Jim's reputation flourished, I grew even more proud of his stature as a national leader. A notable example was when Jim and his wonderful colleagues were recognized on the national TV show *Nightline* a number of years ago. The host Ted Koppel introduced the story of BHCHP by remarking: "Now here's a story that will really make you feel good about yourselves." I remember thinking: "Hey, this is a good deal! Jim and his colleagues do all the work and we get to feel good about ourselves. That's great!!"

But in the end, I concluded that Koppel was right. Through the profound inspiration of their daily example, Jim and his BHCHP colleagues gently nudge us to re-examine the fundamental questions of human existence. How do we live the ordinary life extraordinarily well? What is ultimate, and what is merely important? How should we lead a life that is good, not merely a good life (as Reverend Peter Gomes might ask)? And what gives us value and worth as humans?

The mission of BHCHP, which Jim and his colleagues practice every day with every fiber of their being, is to accept and support people for who they are. Even in the vignettes presented here, you will find that Jim does not judge but only expresses his sense of caring. He accepts that the lesson from these vignettes is to help us all "muse about life's meanings" as we travel through this "maze of mystery and uncertainty." He voices appreciation that the patients protect him from "any hint of complacency or routine." He recognizes that what's important is the human being, not the human doing. He understands that we are all vulnerable and all wounded in our own way. That is the common bond that ties us all together.

Thirty years after the launch of BHCHP, a lot has changed. Most recently, during my service as the Assistant Secretary for Health at the US Department of Health and Human Services, I could view progress from a national perspective. HRSA now funds over 250 Health Care for the Homeless programs. A US Interagency Council on Homelessness currently coordinates nineteen cabinet secretaries and agency heads to tackle national challenges. The Centers for Medicare and Medicaid Services has funded the National Health Care for the Homeless Council to improve care, heighten quality, and lower costs of caring for the homeless population. And through all these developments, the lessons from BHCHP have served as a beacon for the nation.

But despite this progress, one thing that will never change is the need on the streets. This book will return you to that basic theme, time and again. So savor this volume and appreciate this gem. As you read each story and reflect, you will feel more human and more alive. You will be humbled by the people described here and by the lessons they teach us. Thank you Jim and BHCHP for your passion and compassion in serving as pioneers in healing. May you find the strength to continue your blessed work for many more years to come. And thank you for sharing this extraordinary public health journey with us.

With profound respect and admiration,

Howard K. Koh, M.D., M.P.H.
Harvard T.H. Chan School of Public Health
Boston, Massachusetts

Dedication

DR. PHILIP W. BRICKNER

Dr. Philip W. Brickner, the director of the Robert Wood Johnson Foundation's National Health Care for the Homeless Program from 1985 through 1988, inspired and launched the careers of many of us across the country. As the legendary chief of Community Medicine at St. Vincent's Hospital in New York's Greenwich Village, Dr. Brickner and his intrepid teams of doctors, nurses, and social workers began visiting homeless persons in shelters and SROs (single room occupancy hostels) in the 1960s when their emergency room was inundated by people with no access to primary or preventive care.

Dr. Brickner taught us that we can't wait for people struggling to survive without homes to come to us. Rather, we need to venture out and deliver care wherever homeless people gather and feel comfortable. Throughout these years, Dr. Brickner has always been there as our leader and mentor, following our careers with wisdom, wry humor, and selfless devotion. I cherish the hand-written letters of encouragement that came after each success or milestone. Even in the weeks before his death last year, he and his beloved wife Alice continued to send emails urging me to read key books and poems, including Robert Frost's *Two Tramps in Mud Time*. Provocative, densely packed, and difficult to elucidate, the poem concludes with an exhortation to make one's life work a journey that unites passion and love in addressing the desperate needs of so many in our society.

Dr. Philip W. Brickner was an original. He called us to serve the least among us with equal measures of excellence and joy because that is simply the right thing to do. While he insisted fame was as overrated as it was fleeting, these essays and stories are dedicated to his memory.

INTRODUCTION

Medicine That Matters

In Albert Camus' provocative essay, *The Myth of Sisyphus,* the legendary king of Corinth is condemned by the gods to pursue a hopeless and difficult task for all eternity for the sin of cheating death and relishing life. Sisyphus strenuously labors to push a massive boulder to the top of the mountain each day, only to have it roll back to the bottom. Sisyphus is bent but unbroken despite the absurdity of his daily efforts, and Camus ponders what Sisyphus must be thinking during the solitary journey down the mountainside each evening to the plain where his fallen rock awaits.

These stories and essays, written during similar descents in the quiet night hours that punctuate the long days and hectic clinics of these past three decades, attempt to capture a bit of the joy that surprises us while trying to care for the tragic and heroic individuals who struggle courageously against insurmountable odds. Uneven, bumpy, written all too hastily, and dusty from too much time in drawers and boxes, these pieces are arranged chronologically. My hope is that the humanity of each individual emerges. The background of each essay and story is occasionally an historical event but always the unfinished mosaic of the Boston Health Care for the Homeless Program and the wonderful people who have devoted their careers to serving this poor and vulnerable population.

Every life is many days, day after day.
We walk through ourselves, meeting
robbers, ghosts, giants, old men, young
men, wives, but always meeting ourselves.

—James Joyce, *Ulysses*

The Footsoak

AUGUST 1985

A sea of reluctant faces stared intently as I entered the Nurses' Clinic at Pine Street Inn for the first time in early July of 1985, barely two days after finishing my residency in internal medicine at Massachusetts General Hospital (MGH). During the month of June I had served as the senior medical resident in charge of the Bigelow Intensive Care Unit, the bustling hub that cares for the hospital's most complex and desperately ill patients.

Buoyed by the sense of invincibility that accompanies such passages, I strode into New England's oldest and largest shelter, containing over 700 beds and located barely six blocks from the hospital, with a swagger that drew a stern grimace from Barbara McInnis and the other nurses. After four years of medical school and three years of residency, I had thought my training was finally over. My education in homelessness and poverty was just beginning.

This tepid reception by the nurses took me by surprise and left me deflated. Barbara welcomed me to the nation's only independently licensed nursing clinic, begun almost fifteen years earlier by volunteer nurses from the Accident Floor of Boston City Hospital (BCH). Exasperated by the growing number of homeless persons seen emergently for a host of preventable conditions, the nurses resolved to go directly to the shelter to offer timely care and treatment. Barbara, a nurse with the Massachusetts' Department of Public Health, was assigned to Pine Street Inn in 1972 to help with the control of tuberculosis and other infectious diseases. The shelter's clinic flourished over the years, the silence and apparent indifference of hospitals and physicians notwithstanding.

"Pardon our skepticism, but we've been burned too much and don't trust doctors to take good care of our folks. But you will do just fine if you listen to us and do what we say. You'll have to forget much of what you were taught in residency. Nothing changes in the life of a homeless person unless you slow down and take the time to earn trust and develop a lasting relationship. Consistency and presence are essential. Have coffee, play cards, share bits of yourself. Never judge. Remember that people have lived through hell and listen carefully to their stories. With that as bedrock, delivering health care might just be possible."

Each guest was invited into the clinic and addressed by name. Most homeless persons wander our urban landscapes for days without ever hearing someone call them by name, and the response was exuberant. Eyes opened, heads lifted, scowls became smiles.

Virtually all visits to the Nurses' Clinic began with a footsoak.

The waiting area had ten chairs, all occupied by shelter guests soaking their feet in buckets of warm water mixed with an antibacterial called Betadine. This ritual was instituted by the nurses not only for comfort and hygiene, but also as a sign of service and respect. Barbara informed me that my apprenticeship would begin with a couple months of learning the art and skill of soaking feet. She set aside my stethoscope and doctor bag. No medical questions, no chief complaints, no review of systems, no diagnosing.

"Just tend to the feet and ask what else you can do to help."

I dutifully soaked feet for almost two months while observing devoted nurses such as Bob Johansen, Betsy Kendrick, Sheila Healey, Randy Bailey, Mary Hennessey, and so many others, work their magic among weary but grateful pilgrims. In keeping with the obvious biblical allusion, the footsoak inverts the usual power structure and places the caregiver at the feet of each patient and far from the head. This gesture of respect for the literal and figurative personal space of each homeless person is critical and a marked contrast to how I was taught to take charge during clinical encounters, invading privacy each time I placed a stethoscope on the chest, peered at a retina, or examined a throat. After wandering the city for hours, suffering exposure to the extremes of weather, and then standing in a series of queues awaiting entrance to the shelter, a bed ticket, and the evening meal, homeless persons relished the chance to sit and rest while someone cleansed and soothed their feet. I marveled at the overcrowded clinic each evening, teeming with individuals whom we had viewed as intransigent in the hospital and emergency rooms because they repeatedly failed to show up for clinic appointments.

I was 37 years old and finally had my first job as a doctor, although I worried that first night that I should have pursued my oncology fellowship. The journey to medicine was circuitous and serendipitous. I graduated from Notre Dame the spring of the Kent State disaster. Blessed with a high number in the newly instituted draft lottery, I avoided Vietnam and spent two years at Cambridge University in England reading philosophy and theology. The next two years were spent teaching and coaching basketball and track at St. Louis High School in Honolulu, a sojourn in paradise that I will always cherish.

I would have stayed, but I was restless to find my passion, and Hawaii is the most isolated place on the globe, almost 2000 miles from the nearest land in any direction. Listening to the radio in the morning was bizarre as the day's news and events on the mainland were discussed. I had become enamored with the work of Hannah Arendt during my time at Cambridge, and I decided to pursue a doctorate under her direction at the New School in New York City in the fall of 1975. *The Human Condition* had been our bible in college, and her observation on the banality of evil made after attending Eichmann's trial had profoundly influenced me. Her New School seminar on "The Life of the Mind" captivated me and left me spellbound by this strong woman who experienced such history and spoke with conviction and clarity yet conveyed such warm and childlike wonder. But she had a hacking cough which progressed through the fall seminars, and she succumbed to cancer within a few months.

I departed school and returned to work in the Pier Restaurant on the docks of my hometown, Newport, Rhode Island. I had spent summers working there since high school, and I now thought seriously about a career in the restaurant business. Rick Schlegel, my close friend from college who also taught school in Hawaii with me and now worked in the same restaurant, convinced me to save our wages and tips and buy, for a few thousand dollars, an old dairy barn near Smugglers' Notch in northern Vermont. Life there for the next two years was sparse but idyllic, and most of our friends wandered northward and spent time living and skiing with us. I look back on that time as a last gasp of the 1960s, a time when the present was far more important than the future, a time for reading, Socratic dinner discussions, endless skiing on Madonna Mountain, long motorcycle rides, and nurturing friendships while living together hand-to-mouth. I have on occasion lamented we let this all end.

A visit to the Isle of Man upended me. John Orme, my roommate from Cambridge who, after completing his doctorate in engineering, was now a barrister in London, had a home on this beautiful and harsh island, in the middle of the Irish Sea, that hosts an annual Grand Prix motorcycle race. While driving along a narrow, windswept road, the motorcyclist ahead of us was thrown from his bike and badly fractured his lower leg. I sat with this gruff biker from hardscrabble Manchester while John drove to get the volunteer ambulance folks. The conversation during the next 30 minutes ranged from BMWs to a recent divorce to the sexual abuse he endured as a child. Trying not to look at the exposed bone fragments in his leg, I realized that I was profoundly moved and privileged to be sitting with this remarkable man. I only wished that I could have helped with the fractured leg and offered more than a sympathetic ear.

Upon returning home, I went to Brown University to get the basic science courses required for medical school and journeyed back to Vermont each weekend. I wanted to become a country doctor and thought that UVM would be perfect. An admissions counselor winced at my age and said that unless I was "possessed of a font of human energy bordering dangerously on the pathological" he would dissuade me from a career in medicine. I was never invited for the formal interview.

I still harbored the dream of becoming a country doctor when I arrived at Harvard Medical School at the age of 30, but I was soon enraptured by medicine in big city hospitals, chose a residency in medicine at MGH, and planned a career in oncology. In February of my last year, Dr. John Potts, the Chief of Medicine, and Dr. Tom Durant, a mentor and legendary physician who grew up in Dorchester and was devoted to global medicine, called me into the office and asked if I would consider delaying my fellowship for a year to be a full-time doctor for the new health care for the homeless project in Boston. I was savvy enough to recognize a rhetorical question, and I allayed my concerns and embraced this opportunity to ease my late-1960s social conscience with a year of urban Peace Corps. Game on.

Barbara asked me to concentrate on an elderly gentleman with schizophrenia and massively swollen legs. I knew this man well from the MGH emergency room, where he was brought several times a month by EMS. Despite our efforts, he never followed our instructions and refused all medications. The diagnosis in his chart read: "chronic schizophrenia, paranoid type, treatment resistant." His feet were so badly swollen that we needed separate buckets to soak each foot. After about a month, he looked down quizzically at me, smirked, and addressed me for the first time:

"I thought you were supposed to be a doctor. What the hell are you doing soaking my feet?"

Dumbfounded, I couldn't think of anything better to say than, "I do whatever the nurses tell me to do." A few nights later, he told me he was having trouble sleeping at night and would appreciate some help. I remember struggling with how to best respond and offering him a very low dose of the anti-psychotic haloperidol (Haldol), which is quite helpful for sleep. A few days later he came to the clinic and was happy that he was sleeping better, but he asked for a higher dose so that he could sleep longer. Over the next few weeks he opened up to me, accepting my offer of medication to help with his mood and his auditory hallucinations. Three months later he was placed in a group home—after 25 years on the streets and in the shelters. Barbara just smiled, no I-told-you-so's.

I came to this job buoyed to make a difference. Barbara taught us to forget plans—"plans get executed"—and live in the present. She had no pretenses about changing the world and eschewed any titles or leadership roles.

"Follow your heart, just do whatever needs to be done next."

David McGrath, a Navy veteran who worked as a nurse in the clinic in the early 1970s, remembers soaking feet as the portal to the hearts of both patient and clinician. In the midst of changing buckets one night he heard an elderly man who had just come in on a rainy and cold day ask:

"Miss Barbara, why are you so good to us?"

"I'm just being good to your feet right now in case you decide to use them again to get up and walk on out of here."

Soaking feet proved an apt apprenticeship and set the tone for our new program.

Our initial team included Yoshiko Vann, a seasoned and stellar nurse practitioner, and Marc Miletsky, a social worker with improbable patience. We shared in the care of all our patients and conducted all our shelter and hospital clinics together: three nights a week at the 700-bed Pine Street Inn, two evenings at Boston's 500-bed Long Island Shelter, two mornings at BCH, and two afternoons at MGH. Work was difficult and wonderful, and the joy and sustenance we drew from each other was a revelation to me. I wondered why anyone would work any other way, especially in such strenuous situations. Whenever I was on vacation, or Yo was on maternity leave, or Marc home with sick children, our patients would continue to be cared for by team members they knew well.

A gnawing discomfort was hard to ignore during those first weeks. As a resident at a major teaching hospital, I had witnessed how doctors who care for excluded populations soon become marginalized by our own profession. A career path in the care of poor and fragile populations was not viable within our academic medical centers and medical schools. I took this job for a year, understanding that I would then move on to a fellowship in oncology. But watching Barbara and the nurses, patiently earning trust and listening to the stories of people who had so little yet courageously played the impossible hands dealt to them by fate and bad luck, brought unexpected joy and satisfaction accompanied by far more complicated medical challenges than I had ever anticipated. I sensed tumultuous but heady days ahead.

Eyes and Needles

SEPTEMBER 1985

"Where's the Iris Foundation?"
Donald Brooks huddled in the office
doorway early one August Monday in
1985. A diminutive man of forty-eight
years, his forlorn countenance
reminded me of a forgotten teddy
bear—face round and gentle, floppy
cartilaginous ears with wide-set eyes
and broad flattened forehead,
Montgomery monocle tentatively
perched on the left cheekbone, and
tattered Farmer John's beneath an
oversized army surplus jacket.

This camouflaged fatigue coat, suggesting either a desire for obscurity or the intensity of a mission, underscored his painful shyness. He continued as if from a prepared text.

"Kalispell, Montana. I just got off the bus. I live in an abandoned trailer at the far end of Main Street. The neighbors gave me an extension cord so that I can have a light and a hot plate, and the police gave me a television for Christmas last year. I clean up every morning at the diner, and I spend my days in the library. Two weeks ago I lost the vision in my right eye. Everything became blurry and reddish. I've had diabetes since I was a kid, and I know just everything about that disease. One of the magazines I read each week in the library told about bleeding into the iris that can cause a red veil to come over an eye, and I'm sure that has happened to me. In the back of that magazine there was an ad by the Iris Foundation which said they could fix the problem, so I called the number and they told me to come on out here to Boston."

I had arrived two hours early that morning to try and catch up on some charts before clinic began at nine, and I wondered how Mr. Brooks had penetrated the security system. The stench in the tiny room had become oppressive. Three desks and an armchair had been crammed into our office, a former examination room in Boston City Hospital that had no windows. The August heat wave had greeted the sunrise with 85 humid degrees, and the air conditioning had not worked in weeks.

"Mr. Brooks, it's very nice to meet you, and welcome to Boston. Have you found a place to stay?"

"I intend to camp out, Doctor. I buried all of my things in a graveyard across town for safekeeping. The police in Kalispell told me to beware of pickpockets and thieves here in the big city. With my diabetes, I need milk several times a day, and so I bought this half-gallon two days ago and I keep it tied to my belt with this rope."

He opened the plastic bottle and took a sip, demonstrating proudly how the rope offered just enough slack to allow the bottle to reach his mouth. The milk was utterly rancid, and I fought a wave of nausea by forging ahead with questions about his diabetes.

"How much insulin do you take to control your diabetes?"

"Depends. I'll take insulin anywhere from three to eight times a day. I know my body very well and many signals can alert me that my sugar is up and I need more insulin. For example, I often see spots in front of my eyes in the early afternoon. If I take five to ten units of insulin, they're gone in half an hour. Sometimes I feel like I've had two to three cups of coffee, and then I know I need some more insulin. I never touch coffee because it makes my sleeping problems much worse."

"Do you have a lot of trouble sleeping?"

"Since I was a kid. They used to give me pills to slow me down, but I never could fall asleep until after I had been in bed for a couple of hours. Now I just stay up until three or four in the morning and watch the late movies, and even then I still have trouble falling asleep."

"Mr. Brooks, do you have a regular doctor who helps you control your diabetes?"

"Not since I left Detroit."

"How long ago was that?"

"Maybe fifteen years."

"And all this time you've managed to control your diabetes on your own. You've obviously done a very remarkable job. Would you mind if perhaps we could do a bit of a tuneup while you're in town?"

"That's why I'm here, Doctor. I know there's no way this Iris Foundation will take me unless I've been examined by a physician. They told me that over the phone."

"We should also check your blood sugar early some morning before you've eaten anything."

Donald began to fidget in the armchair while shuffling his feet, which barely reached the tile floor.

"No blood tests," he stammered while losing eye contact for the first time since he stepped into the room.

"Do needles bother you?"

"Heavens no. I've been poking myself with needles ever since I can remember. But I've been reading about this plague called AIDS, and I know it comes from dirty needles and big cities. People at the diner warned me about painted ladies, queers, and druggies—all of whom seem to hang out in big cities like Boston. You die if you get AIDS, and you can get it from any of those people. I also know from the magazines I've been reading that you can get AIDS from blood transfusions. So I ain't about to let anyone stick needles into me while I'm here in Boston."

This was the summer of 1985. I was awed by this simple gentleman's understanding and awareness of the coming plague. Even though the world was about to change dramatically, neither Boston nor Kalispell had yet to encounter any known AIDS cases in the homeless community. I was very much concerned about his diabetes, especially because of his probable retinal hemorrhage and his very unorthodox methods of self-treatment for over fifteen years.

"AIDS is indeed a very frightening illness, Mr. Brooks, and I'm again very impressed with your knowledge and understanding. However, the blood tests drawn here in the hospital laboratory are done with needles which are used only once, so there's no danger of contracting the virus. I can assure you of that. But I also know that the ophthalmologists who will fix your eye will for sure require that you have some blood tests done before the surgery."

"I'll have to think about this."

He politely excused himself, muttering that he needed to get to the Public Library at Copley Square by nine. He promised to see me later in the day in the clinic at Pine Street Inn.

Three nights later Donald, tearful and bleeding from several orbital lacerations sustained when someone's fist had shattered his monocle, was assisted into Pine Street Inn. As we dressed and bandaged the wounds—the lacerations were not deep enough to require sutures—he spoke about learning the ways of the city.

"Very frightening out there, very frightening. I tried to sleep in the shelter the first few nights, but all the coughing and snoring kept me awake. I tried to sleep in the Common last night after I made friends with a young couple. They took my wallet while I was asleep, and I haven't seen them since. Today I went into the men's room at

Filene's and tried to wash up, but some high school kids called me trash and pushed me into one of the stalls. I slipped and fell against the toilet and broke my glass. They just laughed. Without the glass I'm just about blind, and I had to ask for help getting back here to the shelter. The police just dropped me off."

He didn't feel much like talking, but he agreed to take a bed in the shelter for the night. The staff found him some clean clothes, although he refused to part with the cincture and a newly purchased half gallon of Cumberland Farms milk.

The Iris Foundation was actually the Retina Foundation, and we made an appointment for an evaluation at the Eye and Ear Infirmary. He reluctantly agreed to come to see me at the Massachusetts General Hospital clinic for the pre-operative physical examination and the dreaded blood tests. He insisted I draw the blood myself, and to my utter surprise his blood glucose was minimally elevated and his other laboratory results were normal. His examination was notable only for signs of diabetic retinopathy in the left eye. I was unable to see anything other than blood in the right eye.

Donald spoke reticently about himself. Born in 1937 on a farm in Kansas, he was the youngest of nine children. Times were difficult, and the family moved several times to unsuccessful farms in Illinois and Michigan, forcing several of the children to be placed in foster homes. Donald managed to finish the eighth grade but ran away after he was physically and sexually abused by his foster parents. He took odd jobs as a laborer and later went on to get his high school equivalency degree. He married at age 27, fathered three daughters, and supported his family as a roofer and carpenter in the Detroit area. Divorce ended the marriage in 1979 for reasons he chose not to share with me or perhaps never understood. A few days before he returned to Kalispell that fall, he admitted that he had always had troubles "with the nerves" and had been hospitalized several times in Detroit and placed on medications which made him feel "out to lunch" so he refused to take them. He had hitchhiked to the West after the divorce and had been in Kalispell since 1981. He had no contact with his family, and he was pretty sure that his daughters had no idea where he was.

"Mr. Brooks, how have you gotten your insulin through the years without a prescription?"

"Oh, I got a prescription when I left Detroit. The pharmacist in town has always refilled my insulin whenever I've run out. I have to leave it in the refrigerator at the diner most of the time, though."

"What about the needles and syringes?"

"Those are easy to get, and besides, one syringe will last me a couple of months at least. Let me show you."

From the pocket of his camouflage jacket he pulled a yellowed tabloid newspaper and carefully unrolled it. He withdrew an insulin syringe, or so it seemed. The unit markings and numbers were worn away, and the needle was bent at a 45 degree angle and rotated easily on the long axis of the syringe. Donald's fear of communicable viruses had led him to use his own needles over and over again. Repeated punctures of the skin with used needles, especially ones wrapped in dirty newspapers, would likely cause horrible infections in diabetics; but once again, I was a newcomer in a world of survivors, and their game was played by other rules. I spoke sheepishly about the importance of using needles only once, but Donald looked askance and maintained a polite demeanor as he carefully wrapped the syringe in the same newspaper.

The operation went very well, although the pre- and post-operative care was challenging. The surgeons initially refused to do the delicate eye surgery unless we could assure them that Donald would have a safe and stable place to receive post-operative care. To maximize healing, he would have to lie horizontal and remain as still as possible for two weeks—virtually impossible for a person living on the streets or in the shelters. Standing, sitting, and lifting were all forbidden. So Donald became one of the first patients admitted to our medical respite unit that opened in September. This was the first in the country but soon was followed by the remarkable Christ House in Washington, D.C. Our 25-bed unit was nested within the 100-bed state-run Shattuck Shelter, adjacent to the Lemuel Shattuck Hospital and Boston's Franklin Park, the gem of Frederick Law Olmsted's "Emerald Necklace" of interconnected parks and pathways linking the Charles River to the Dorchester Basin.

The creation of a medical respite unit was a mandate of the community coalition that raged against the policy of hospitals prematurely discharging homeless persons who did not have a place in which to heal and have family, VNA, and other supportive services. The goal was to offer 24-hour medical and nursing care to homeless persons too ill or medically compromised to withstand the daily rigors of life on the streets but not so sick as to require costly acute-care hospitalization. Donald was an ideal candidate and was admitted just a few weeks after he first appeared in the office. We had earned just enough trust to win his begrudging acceptance. We allowed him to keep his own milk, administer his own insulin with clean needles he reluctantly accepted, and refuse any blood tests. He grew fond of Betty Snead, our first respite aide, who bantered and cajoled and laughed with him each evening during her 3PM to 11PM shift. Our clinical staff, including myself, would seek Betty's intercession with any request we had of Donald. This reminded me repeatedly that each member of our team served an essential and invaluable role.

Donald was the harbinger of a world about to change. During that autumn, dozens of poor and homeless individuals living in shelters and on the streets were diagnosed with AIDS. Our respite unit was soon overwhelmed with individuals suffering the ravages of the many opportunistic infections and neoplasms. We had no effective treatments, and death stalked daily as countless homeless men and women succumbed, often estranged from family and loved ones, alone and lonely.

Within a month Donald had recovered virtually all of the vision in his right eye and left our respite unit to return to his campsite along the Muddy River. After passing his six-week post-operative check with flying colors, he stopped by the office and bade me farewell. He said I could write to him on Main Street in Kalispell, which I did that Christmas, but he never answered.

Epidemics of Hopelessness

JANUARY 1986

BHCHP was forged from the crucible of tuberculosis and AIDS, two epidemics that devastated Boston's homeless population in the mid-1980s and dramatically shaped our care-delivery model while immeasurably complicating our clinical lives. In addition to caring for individual patients, I was soon catapulted headlong into the world of public health and communicable diseases.

Still anxious to impress the shelter nurses with my clinical acumen, I carefully examined a man in the lobby of Pine Street Inn in August of 1985 who "just didn't look right" to the shelter staff. A heavy smoker and longstanding drinker, ebullient and boisterous, frustrated by all the unwanted attention, he insisted he was fine. He was afebrile, and his heart and lungs were unremarkable on examination with my stethoscope. I told the nurses and the lobby staff that I couldn't find anything acutely wrong, but I asked them to keep an eye on him and be sure to bring him back to clinic if their concerns persisted. Two days later he was brought in, and we obtained a chest x-ray that showed advanced cavitary tuberculosis, a condition commonly seen in third-world settings but not often just a few blocks from three academic medical centers.

In the mid-1980s, more than 60 individuals sleeping at the shelter contracted pulmonary tuberculosis, with over half of the cases involving a multi-drug-resistant organism. Each person needed four medications a day for eighteen months, a daunting task that taught us the value of partnerships (state and city departments of public health, shelters, hospitals, community health centers) and the necessity of working as a team (with the doctor often the least important member). Dr. John Bernardo, a pulmonologist at Boston City Hospital who specializes in tuberculosis, and Dr. Ed Nardell of the Massachusetts Department of Public Health came several times each week to the shelter to work with Barbara McInnis, the other nurses, and our team to identify and treat those with active tuberculosis as well as those exposed to the organism in the shelter.

Many who contracted tuberculosis fled to the streets, afraid to return to the shelter where they became sick. Our first efforts at "street medicine" in 1985 involved venturing out each day to find our patients and observe them taking their medications on park benches, down back alleys, along the Charles River. Over 90% of these people completed the full treatment course, and thankfully no one died from tuberculosis, a remarkable affirmation of the efforts of an extraordinary team working together with the state and city departments of public health.

One month after we saw our patient with cavitary tuberculosis, a man who had been angrily evicted by his partner from their South End apartment came to see us at the clinic at Pine Street Inn. He had massively swollen legs that were discolored by Kaposi's sarcoma. He was the first person known to be diagnosed with AIDS in a Boston shelter. Panic and dread gripped the shelter community in the wake of this poorly understood and deadly virus. Hastily called late-night staff meetings were boisterous and vituperative as the details of AIDS were discussed, with raging arguments over the use of common toilets, the necessity of separate showering and shaving facilities, the need to quarantine those infected, and even whether those with AIDS should be allowed to use the shelter. The irony was inescapable, as the shelters, with their prevalence of tuberculosis, infestations, and other communicable diseases, were far more dangerous places for those whose immune systems were destroyed by AIDS. We found ourselves pleading, usually without much success in those early days, with hospitals and jails not to discharge persons with AIDS to the shelters.

The complexity and urgency of the daily clinical work necessitated by these two epidemics was overwhelming as we also endeavored to create and implement a health care service-delivery model for homeless individuals and families that offered high quality, accessible, and continuous care. Care in the ICU seemed straightforward in comparison. In the days before effective anti-retroviral treatment, AIDS was a virtual death sentence, and the circumstances of those deaths among homeless persons with AIDS were often horrifying and are indelibly etched in my memory. One of my first patients to die of AIDS had been previously healthy but suddenly began acting bizarrely in Long Island Shelter and developed a fever and headache. A neurologist in the emergency room carefully examined him, wrote in the chart that our patient was "malingering," and discharged him to the streets. Two days later, this 32-year-old man was found dead in the back of an abandoned car. The autopsy revealed Herpes encephalitis related to AIDS as the cause of death.

Our 25-bed medical respite unit at the Lemuel Shattuck Shelter became primarily an AIDS unit as we struggled to treat infections and other complications of this virus as best we could. By December 1985, seven individuals were diagnosed with AIDS, and no one lived longer than nine months before they succumbed to *Pneumocystis carinii* pneumonia, Kaposi's sarcoma, or any of the myriad other opportunistic infections with debilitating consequences such as blindness or dementia. People literally wasted away before us, and our tools were primitive, leaving us feeling inadequate and devastated as we witnessed so many suffer and die alone and lonely, without so much as the dignity of a home or a family.

Morning Clinic,
Boston City Hospital
AUGUST 1986

I have come to cherish the dark and
peaceful hours after midnight, when
details of daily routine succumb to
musings about life's meaning and the
moral and ethical assumptions that
guide our personal and professional
journeys through this maze of mystery
and uncertainty. Sporadic attempts
to write some notes have been all too
feeble, with stories more often dangling
than complete. Yet the yearning and
need to write reflects an attempt to
make some sense of these days and
years that are given to us.

Answers have been hard to come by. I remember years ago reading Paul of Samosata, a second-century philosopher who was bewildered by religious wars and hatred. He noted that each of the world's great religions required a lifetime of devotion, sacrifice, faith, and study to fully comprehend. Yet each human being was given but a single life, making it impossible to ever know for sure whether one had chosen the right road. When someone asked me today why I do this work, I shrugged my shoulders, offered a few empty platitudes, and waited until tonight to find a minute to think about it. And now I feel particularly vulnerable, and I've been reading through the notes from this morning's clinic.

I opened the office at Boston City Hospital at 7AM. The walls have been whitewashed of windows and posters, and I'm embarrassed to think we've been content with such blandness for so long. I managed to complete several SSI forms that had cluttered my desktop for weeks. Pat Sullivan, the wonderful nurse practitioner at Long Island Shelter, called to let me know about several crises over the weekend. Clifford Roswell was sent into the emergency room with multiple stab wounds, thankfully all superficial. James Williamson had a probable pneumonia and needed to have his chest x-ray reviewed. The shelter staff was shattered by Rick Gifford's unexpected death last Thursday. Rick had chronic heart failure and had been on dialysis for a decade with end-stage renal disease. He had been increasingly agitated, and last Wednesday night he had been in a fight with Donald Nestor over some racial slurs. That episode caused him to be barred from the shelter, and we decided to admit him to the VA Hospital in Jamaica Plain. We had to finesse the system, as Rick was *persona non grata* on the wards. Apparently he had hospitalized a staff member with his cane several years ago, and in his chart he was noted to be "irreparable and incorrigible" and had to be accompanied by two guards at all times while on the VA grounds. But now he was very short of breath, unable to return to the shelter he cherished, and the VA folks admitted Rick "for observation." The next morning he had a cardiac arrest and died. He was 44 years old. The shelter staff agonized because the death of this beloved guest followed the barring. Long Island had been his only home during the last three years of his life.

Yoshiko Vann arrived soon after I hung up. Having spent the previous two weeks with her family on the New Jersey coast, she was definitely not looking forward to the specter of Monday clinic ahead. Tall, elegant, black and Japanese, Yo was our nurse practitioner. A legendary outreach nurse for the city's TB clinic for many years and skilled in karate, Yo was a wizard on the streets—conniving, caring, cajoling, flirting. I remember one psychotic gentleman who had called the office during a blizzard last winter, asking if we would dispatch some soup and warm blankets on the Yoshiko "van," presumably confusing Yoshiko with Pine Street's overnight van or Kit Clark's meal truck. We commiserated well into the second cup of coffee, realizing that this was also our first day without Dargis Valdez. A native of Santo Domingo, Dargis was our extraordinary team coordinator who kept our lives almost organized. She had a falling out with our director and gave her notice; unfortunately no one had yet been found to replace her.

Marc Miletsky arrived last, after spending the night moonlighting at The Arbor, a psychiatric hospital in Jamaica Plain. A social worker and veteran of the glory days of Berkeley, Marc has improbable patience with his impossible job. An astute critic and philosopher of both guilt and race, he had been the first to notice what a collage our team was: Caribbean Hispanic, Black Japanese, New York Jewish, and Irish Catholic. My first-ever shot as a minority.

Dorothy Dexter knocked and entered the office without waiting for an answer at 8:15AM, having arrived on the morning van from Pine Street Inn. Homeless for as many years as anyone could remember, Dorothy proudly wore a scar from her left ear all the way around to the middle of her right cheek. Despite the fact that I had spent a full year caring for Dorothy's hypertension and obstructive lung disease, the history behind the scar remained a mystery shrouded by an elegant paranoia. This morning Dorothy sat in the chair, pocketbook resting on her lap, posture utterly erect, and detailed several symptoms suggesting an upper respiratory infection which had plagued her over the weekend. She then sat back and awaited my examination and diagnosis. I have learned to be painstaking and restrained in my dealings with Dorothy; she always threw down the gauntlet and sat with noble but demanding patience while I performed the perfunctory role of the doctor. Her lungs sounded perfectly clear, temperature was normal, her sputum appeared benign under the microscope. I then explained to Dorothy that I felt she most likely had a viral infection of the upper respiratory tract. After detailing the ineffectiveness of antibiotics for viruses, I wrote a prescription for an over-the-counter decongestant which she would then be able to purchase with her Medicaid card. Presenting the script to Dorothy, I completed the ritual. She grumbled brusquely, catching my eyes for a millisecond as she stood, and headed off for another week. Dorothy is unique, and I had come to accept and admire her ingratitude. That horrible scar bespoke a violence which had undoubtedly given her reason to flee into the nightmare of paranoia—yet somehow Dorothy Dexter salvaged her dignity in the dogged protection of that secret which belonged only to herself. As such she had come to eschew charity and handouts, and she truly expected and deserved to be given a measure of excellence in her medical care.

The waiting room we shared with the patients of the hospital's busy Medical Walk-in Clinic was bustling and noisy, and Monday was in full swing. I tried to call the next patient, but four or five jumped up and came to offer urgent pleas. My eye caught a very distraught and tremulous Jeff Noonan sitting on the floor in front of the large glass wall overlooking Massachusetts Avenue. I went over to see what was happening, and no one seemed to object when I brought him into the examining room.

Jeff had first come to see me months ago, shortly after discovering that he had tested positive for HIV. To him this was a death sentence, and he was having a very difficult time coping. After graduating from Malden High School as a three-letter star athlete, he joined the Army during the Vietnam era. To his chagrin he was given a tour in Spain and never saw action or Southeast Asia. After a transfer to California near the end of his stint with the Army, he mingled with several Vietnam combat vets and was introduced to intravenous drugs. This escalated rapidly to a $200–300 per day habit. He lost interest in all else, and for seventeen years he relentlessly pursued the only thing he ever really wanted.

Ruggedly handsome and an imposing 6' 4" tall, Jeff was an Irish charmer who came from a family of six children. His father and uncle were Malden firemen. He spoke often of wanting to somehow win his father's respect but frequently came to the office crying over disastrous attempts at reconciliation. In the mid-1970's, after he had been told to never again return home, he retaliated by taking a shotgun and firing point blank into his abdomen, splattering his spleen and perforating his small intestine. As he sheepishly admitted, he never wanted to kill himself but rather just mutilate and maim.

A younger cousin had been his closest friend, and in some contorted gesture to help her escape a failing marriage, he introduced her to heroin and life on the streets. A year ago February she was found raped and killed in a back alley of Portland, Maine. Two nights later a high school friend of hers was found dead near the same alley. The killer, a psychiatric escapee from New Hampshire, was apprehended in a white van that same week. Jeff never recovered from that loss, and to himself and his entire family he was forever guilty of his cousin's murder. We had talked about this for a long time last winter, and I recall the unspeakable horror in his eyes as he pulled a tattered newspaper from his pocket and cursed himself and the world for the prurient headlines eulogizing his beloved cousin and best friend: "Naked Woman Found Raped and Strangled in Dumpster."

Six weeks ago Jeff had a major battle with his father. He had known that his positive HIV serology would be incomprehensible and intolerable for his Dad, and he had shared the news only with his mother. By a simple clerical error at the VA, an announcement of a study available to all HIV seropositive patients was inadvertently sent to Jeffrey, Sr. It was the last straw in their relationship.

"You'd be better off dead than being my son."

Jeff headed for Chelsea to stay with some friends and quickly got himself arrested for shoplifting several bottles of Tylenol worth two to three dollars each on the street. Jeff had explained to me some time ago how one could support a large heroin habit by shoplifting innocuous items worth less than $50, assuring only a misdemeanor if caught. Jeff had no bail and spent the night locked up. He was found the following morning hanging by his belt in his cell, appearing cyanotic but still breathing. Rushed to Whidden Hospital, he suffered a respiratory arrest en route and was successfully resuscitated in the emergency room. After a week in the ICU, he was transferred to a psychiatric facility on the North Shore, where he had been for the past two weeks.

This morning he appeared exhausted and cachectic, but his mind was characteristically sharp and incisive.

"I guess I don't need to ask you why, Jeff."

"It's just too much. This god dammed death sentence is just too much to handle. I have no family, my friends have deserted me, I can't even sleep with my girlfriend without thinking I'm about to kill her. I've been cursed all my life and now the curse is literally running through my blood. I'm addicted to drugs and I realize I'll never shake it. But heck, why would I quit now? But it's funny, I'm slowly coming to grips with who I am, and I know clearly that I've just been along for the ride all these years. I've never contributed anything. I've never taken control of anything in my life."

Jeff had no signs or symptoms of AIDS or AIDS Related Complex (ARC), and persons in his situation at that time fell into a netherworld of uncertainty. While it was likely that he would become ill, we still were not sure how many persons with the virus would actually contract clinical AIDS. Jeff didn't buy that. He had been told that since he had lost his spleen he was at greater risk for developing opportunistic infections. And he had destroyed his own spleen with a shotgun blast, almost in prophetic preparation for the virus through which reparation and salvation would be wrought. The writing was on the wall.

"The only war I've ever waged has been against my own body and my own cursed genes, and I've done a damn good job."

Jeff admitted that he had resumed both heroin and cocaine as soon as he had been discharged from the psychiatric facility yesterday afternoon. He still shared his needles most of the time. I didn't argue or judge this day, but I did press him on why he continued to put others at risk.

"All addicts have a death wish. We are all enslaved by our habits, and the thought that some virus hidden in our needles might finally release us can be welcomed and embraced during those horrible moments of drug sickness before the next dose. But don't worry, Doc, I know that there's nothing you can offer and I don't blame you a bit."

I was deeply concerned.

Three weeks later, on August 31, Jeff cashed his SSI check, left a note for his girlfriend, and injected enough heroin to end his war and declare a separate and final peace.

Walter Tibbles' blood pressure was under good control with the new once-daily medication we had obtained from a drug company, and Marc and I celebrated his first SSI check. Walter had an IQ of 58, had never learned to read or write, and couldn't tell time. At our first meeting in March, I was dumbfounded as I spoke with this sweet and gentle human being who had few of the skills necessary for survival in our society. A stammering, crescendo stutter had shielded his disability through years of menial jobs cleaning toilets, mopping floors, and scouring pots and pans. Through his 35 years, he had been scorned and scapegoated and had turned to alcohol for some small measure of self-confidence. Somewhere lost in time, he had been labeled a drunk and fallen through all the cracks in the system. We had written long letters, and Marc had walked Walter through the SSI system, and within weeks he had received a check and was now about to move into a room of his own in Springfield near his family.

Ida Timms was next. She had stopped by for blood tests. We had admitted her for *Pneumocystis carinii* pneumonia in early July, and she had recovered rapidly, although she did not endear herself to the nursing staff when she was found sharing needles in the bathroom. We worked closely with the newly formed AIDS Clinic at the hospital, and Ida was later to be among the first patients at Boston City Hospital to begin AZT. She had to take her pills every four hours around the clock, which meant that the counselors at Long Island Shelter would have to awaken her at 2AM each night. Ida embodied the challenge to the homeless community to learn to care for those with AIDS who faced overwhelming addictions and almost certain death without having a place to live.

Eric Bachelor came to have his blood sugar checked and to get some help with a housing form. Charlotte Devine, with a chartreuse wig and mauve miniskirt, needed refills of her cardiac medications somewhat early. She cashed her monthly SSI check and bought a discount ticket to London, where she intended to live on a houseboat on the Thames. Hypomanic and histrionic, Charlotte maintained a separate conversation with her voices during my examination of her heart and lungs. She riled when I suggested she might speak to the psychiatric nurse downstairs. Alberto Navarro followed, wearing his usual respiratory mask to protect his lungs from the pollution of Boston, and muffled:

"Marriage is a matter of temperature, not temperament."

I have no idea what he meant by that, but it does make one think. Tortured by an obsessive-compulsive disorder, Alberto craves cleanliness. I have learned patience with his hypochondriasis, and Dante's description of the Inferno pales in comparison with Alberto's diatribes about living amidst the infestations and filth in the shelters. No worse a hell-on-earth can be imagined for someone like Alberto.

Clinic ran well into the afternoon, punctuated by the flurry of calls to and from the shelter clinics, welfare agencies, and detoxification units. After some frantic paperwork, the three of us headed for our evening clinic at Pine Street Inn. We finished around 9:30PM, and our team limped to join Barbara McInnis and the other nurses for a beer at Doyle's Pub in Jamaica Plain.

These are the lives I've stumbled upon. Not orderly or reasoned, and not the way lives are supposed to be. Many would challenge the patience of Job and make us wonder whether any loving God would allow such serendipity. Lives with more questions than answers, lives shrouded in the mysteries of fate and genetics. But as I write now into the early morning hours, I find richness and a fulfillment I can't quite explain. I have always had an irrational fear of boredom and ennui, and these wonderfully erratic pilgrims have protected me from any hint of complacency or routine.

Free Wheeling

NOVEMBER 1986

Early last month, Marc Miletsky called
from across the hall in our Boston
City Hospital clinic to introduce me to
Bob Grauer. This 35-year-old Vietnam
veteran had just arrived in town via
wheelchair from Nashville.
He had been told to come to see us
because we might be able to help
him fix the bent wheel of his chair.
An eighteen-wheeler had "dusted me"
on Interstate 95, rendering the rim
of his right wheel sinusoid.

Bob wore a ten-gallon Stetson, flannel shirt glittering with colorful buttons, and alligator boots with large holes in both soles. The Army fatigues were frayed and tattered. He was unshaven and delightfully hypomanic.

"Rhymes with 'Power,'" he chortled as he introduced himself to me.

Marc had just weathered an hour with Bob and was spent. I agreed to see Bob that evening at our Pine Street Inn Clinic, and in the meantime we'd see about finding a spare wheel for his chair.

Just after he finished dinner at the shelter, Bob barreled into clinic, and we had some time to talk. The reasons for his left-sided paralysis were not at all clear, and I was anxious to find them out. The wheelchair was a sight. In addition to the severely bent rim, seven or eight spokes were missing, and the rubber tire had been virtually worn through to the metal rim. Bob carefully explained that he had begun his marathon journey eight years ago in Hyannis, and over 28 months he had zigzagged his way across the country to San Diego. Since then he had done the transcontinental route four times, and most recently he had been in Nashville. His technique was unusual. He didn't use the smaller roads, instead preferring the interstate highways. The paralysis of his left arm and leg meant that it was easier to wheel backward.

"Those semi's will catch you in their draughts and make the wheeling easy. I can crank out 60-70 miles a day in good weather."

"I tried to confiscate a wheelchair from the hospital after I saw you guys today, but I couldn't get away fast enough. They wouldn't accept any trade-ins. Up until eight years ago I was happily married. My wife balled my best friend and decided he was a better lay. Thank God, they also decided to take the kids with them. All thirteen of them! That poor bastard is now saddled with thirteen kids and that bitch. They sold my ranch near Boise and kept every single dime. I didn't get a thing."

"Do you get any VA benefits, Mr. Grauer?"

"They don't give a fuck about me, and I don't give a fuck about them. I was in St. Mary's Hospital in Long Beach, California, about six years ago and President Reagan was bragging about increasing the pensions for all veterans. National TV was there, and I took my Medal of Honor and I told him to stuff it up his you-know-where and rotate. Everybody cheered me on, but ever since then I've been cut off from all my VA benefits."

Bob said he had grown up as a Navy brat and was in a different city and different school each year. Apparently he had done very well, although he enlisted in the Marines as soon as he turned eighteen.

"I joined the Marines as soon as I was old enough, and I couldn't wait to get over to Vietnam. My father was a captain in the Navy, and it was my goal in life to show him up. I was a kid in a garden of wonder, carrying guns and shooting up gooks, and there were wonderful women and drugs everywhere you turned. I tried everything, but mostly heroin. I was always in trouble, mostly because I insisted on wearing my ten-gallon over my beret. Fuck 'em if they can't take a joke! But I got shot up pretty bad in this left leg in 1967, and I was a POW for several months until I escaped with two buddies. At Da Nang I got right back into the fighting and took a shitload of shrapnel in my chest and head. Just about half my head was hanging in the breeze, so I put on the Stetson to keep everything in place and kept fighting like hell. When the fighting was over the Marines were evacuating Da Nang and I was in some hospital having a subdural hematoma evacuated from my head. I've never been able to use my left leg or my left arm since."

"Now I get off on busting up my father. He'll panic when he finds out I'm back in the area, and I'm sure he'll give me enough money to get back out West. Then I'll find some new towns and bust them up a bit too. Whenever I show up I can usually get everybody all riled and confused and feeling sorry for me. It's a blast."

And that's exactly what happened. Marc miraculously found a new wheel, and Bob's parents wired him a ticket to Oklahoma City for the following week.

"Who the hell wants to go to Oklahoma City?"

We never saw Bob again. The dim world between fact and fiction seemed to be his special frontier, and his mania brought blinding floodlights to that netherworld. Marc and I had marveled at the vision of this modern-day cowboy with boots and Stetson riding his wheelchair backwards down the highways of America and leaving silver bullets in the shelters and soup kitchens at the crossroads he so dramatically disrupted.

Long Island Shelter

NOVEMBER 1987

Lucretia Harvey was stabbed on
Long Island in late November of 1987.
May Reid, a resident in medicine at
Massachusetts General Hospital, had
come with me that Thursday afternoon
to visit Long Island Shelter, a public
facility for 450 men and women
situated on an island in the midst
of Boston's ignominious harbor—
the country's most polluted according
to the Environmental Protection
Agency, a fact that later became
an acerbic issue in George Bush's
defeat of Michael Dukakis in
the 1988 Presidential Campaign.

Despite the first snow of the season and the usual Southeast Expressway melee, the ten-mile trek from Boston City Hospital was unevent-
ful, and we arrived on time for the weekly clinic meeting. I looked forward to this gathering of the nursing and social service staff as a time
of commiseration, sharing, and rejuvenation; a time when difficult
problems are discussed and workable treatment plans are organized.
May's ebullient questioning was refreshing, and the staff's answers
underscored the competence and dedication of these caregivers.

Just after 3:30PM, the first bus arrived, and the clinic doors
opened to the usual frenzy that marks life before bed assignments
and dinner. The shelter had been opened by the City of Boston in
1983 in response to the escalating numbers and visibility of homeless
persons. Neighborhoods were reluctant to embrace such a large influx
of indigents, and the NIMBY (not-in-my-back-yard) issues were skirt-
ed by converting the former tuberculosis sanatorium adjacent to the
city's Chronic Disease Hospital on Long Island into a 450-bed shelter.
Homeless persons gathered at Boston City Hospital each afternoon
and were bussed from 3PM to 7PM to the Island, where a hot meal and
bunk beds awaited them.

Duke's urgent voice called from one of the far corridors:

"Doctor! The women's bathroom, come quickly!"

The floor counselors are seasoned, and such panic seldom punc-
tuates their entreaties. I bolted to the bathroom with May and Joan
McMahon, the head nurse, a few yards behind.

"Something's happened to young Lucretia, and there's blood all
over the place," stuttered Duke in a muted monotone. I had never
learned his surname, an exasperating but charming aspect of the
streets, where first names more than suffice and titles are largely ignored. Born in Haiti, Duke had been an invaluable support to several
of his homeless country folk who suffered from AIDS. He not only
translated Creole but also helped us understand the torment and hu-
miliation of such cultural and social isolation.

The crowd, clustered on the threshold of the bathroom, parted
to let us run through. A pervasive silence bespoke the severity of the

situation. In the shelter, noise is reassuring, silence dreadful. Lucretia Harvey was writhing on the floor in front of the far stall.

"Lucretia, what hurts?"

I knelt beside this 60-year-old woman who had been at the shelter with her daughter for over two years. Eyes rolled back and pounding her chest in agony, she wailed uncontrollably. Earlier in the year she had complained of severe intermittent chest pain which might well have been angina, but an exercise tolerance test and 24-hour ambulatory electrocardiogram were entirely normal, and we suspected that her pain was caused by severe stress and anxiety. This evening Lucretia couldn't answer me through her gurgles and chortles, but she managed to grab my arm and motion toward the far stall.

Marion Norman, blood dripping from the knife in her right hand, leaned bemusedly against the sink adjacent to the stall. Less than five feet tall, but well over two hundred pounds, this powerful woman had brooding and ferocious eyes. We knew little of her history, as she had chosen to remain mute during interviews. She smiled politely and pointed to Lucretia's pale and whimpering daughter, sitting on the toilet with her clothes clumped at the ankles. Lucretia's daughter, who shared her mother's name, had been stabbed several times, and jets of pulsating arterial blood had reddened the walls and ceiling.

"Please don't let me die, Doctor!"

Young Lucretia 's blood pressure was barely detectable, and May helped me get her to the floor. A deep slash from the neck to the left shoulder had severed the subclavian artery, which was gushing freely. May managed to control that artery while I worked to occlude the left temporal artery, which had been splayed by a gash to the side of the face and which continued to splash bright red blood over us. A third knife wound had fileted the back of Lucretia's left hand, presenting us with a vivid anatomy lesson of the extensor tendons but thankfully not requiring any emergent attention. The shelter's emergency equipment did not include any intravenous medicines, and we could only apply pressure to each of the bleeding points while waiting for the EMTs. During the intensity of such moments of ritualistic response, reason often detours, and I caught myself noting that men virtually always use knives to stab or penetrate deeply, creating small and imperceptible incisions with frequently fatal internal wounds. Women tend to slash, causing very bloody wounds and leaving long disfiguring scars.

Young Lucretia was mentally challenged and had been cared for exclusively by her mother, who had refused to allow formal psychiatric evaluation or testing after her daughter's twenty-first birthday. Both had been physically and sexually abused by the father/husband, and both harbored a deep distrust of men and social service agencies. I had never seen them further than ten feet apart, and this symbiotic relationship had blossomed within the turmoil and danger of the streets. Each was the other's protector and *raison d'être*. They passed entire days together in Boston City Hospital's lobby, and on the bus back to the Island they were inseparable. Words were hardly ever exchanged between them, as if any important issues had long since been exhaustively dissected and resolved. I would often join them for a cup of coffee in the hospital cafeteria and enjoy lively but disparate conversations, as mother and daughter spoke easily with me but never with each other.

Greg Harvey also lived in the shelter, but he avoided his mother and sister and only begrudgingly acknowledged his kinship. He was embarrassed by the inevitable jokes about his sister "the ugly retard" and by the gnarled and matted hairpiece of "Mother Medusa" precariously perched on the brow of his mother's forehead and shimmering with all manner of creature. Suffering from a severe learning disability, Greg was also unable to read or write but proudly worked each day in the labor pool for minimum wages. Fate had dealt him a losing hand, and his chances of escaping the streets were zero. Early in the winter he had come to the hospital clinic with a high fever and was diagnosed with pneumonia. I convinced him to let us care for him in our Medical Respite Unit for a couple of days. He asked if I would call his boss at the labor pool and explain why he would not be able to work. I offered Greg the phone, but he handed it back to me along with the handwritten number on a crumpled piece of scrap paper. He was too humiliated to let me know that he couldn't read numbers or dial phones.

Another daughter had agreed to take them in about a year ago as a result of a monumental effort by several agencies, although three months later mother and young Lucretia fled again to the streets with accusations of neglect and abuse against the daughter's live-in boyfriend, who dealt cocaine in Springfield and found the litigious mother and daughter to be a liability.

Young Lucretia was sobbing, acutely embarrassed by her filth and nakedness. Marion had attacked her while she was defecating, and the admixture of blood, urine, and excrement had smeared her skin and soiled her clothes. The plummeting pressure due to the loss of blood had left her consciousness addled, and she felt no pain. The EMTs arrived after twenty interminable minutes, and mother and daughter were whisked to Boston City Hospital's emergency room. Marion was arrested and sent to Bridgewater for a long-overdue psychiatric evaluation, although she was back on the streets three months later.

The incident had been the result of a longstanding feud between Marion and the two Harvey women over the front seats on the evening bus. During the brief Harvey sojourn in Springfield, Marion had laid claim to one of the front seats previously claimed by the Harveys. Upon returning several weeks ago, Lucretia and her daughter flummoxed Marion by queuing several hours early to ensure access to those seats. The front seats held no particular advantage, other than pride of position. Sometimes that is all that's left.

The packed waiting room of the clinic was eerily quiet and somber, as often happens after such frightening occurrences. The staff was visibly shaken, and Joan ventured a nervous comment on how truth can sometimes be stranger than fiction. Jerry Niles, back in the shelter after a two-week drinking binge and soaking the remnants of his frostbitten feet in a bucket of warm water and Betadine, looked up with an insouciant smile:

"Piece of cake. Fiction, my friends, has to make sense."

A Good Death

MAY 1988

Death lurks steadfastly on the streets and in the shelters. The causes are legion and complex: exposure to the extremes of weather and temperature, the spread of communicable diseases such as tuberculosis and pneumonia in crowded shelters with inadequate ventilation, neglected chronic illnesses, horrifying violence, co-occurring medical and psychiatric illnesses amidst the ravages of substance abuse, and inadequate nutrition, to name only a few. Boston's shelters often hold services for deceased guests, with a funeral and burial arranged when family or next-of-kin are unknown.

Often the person who dies has given us only a street name, leaving us without a way to contact family or loved ones. Many homeless persons prefer to remain anonymous, and we have learned to beware of street names that consist of two first names, such as John Thomas and Robert James, or resemble a beverage or cocktail, such as Tom Collins, Jack Daniels, or Rob Roy. We have come to accept that persons struggling to cope in the shelters and on the streets have been through major life traumas or harbor deep remorse and shame and choose to remain obscure. I often wonder how many families have lost touch with loved ones who are now buried in unmarked graves in paupers' fields somewhere in America.

The services are profoundly moving and are attended by friends, staff, and caregivers, as well as homeless persons from the shelters and the streets. Forgotten souls, weary denizens of America's streets and alleys, forsaken by reason or luck, are afforded the dignity of a memorial service, a belated chance to be recognized, and a final permanent resting place of their own. Unruly drinkers and unkempt street-dwellers wash, shave, don ill-fitting suits gathered from the clothing room, and attend a service to remember one of their own. Proud pallbearers are chosen, and guests are usually transported by van to the church and the graveyard. Tears flow from places long fallow, while the presence of death becomes a gentle and almost soothing reminder of our ultimate equality and destiny.

Four hundred people attended John Hennessy's funeral at Christ the King Church in Woburn last week. Bill Mullen, a remarkable volunteer at the Catholic Worker's Haley House in the South End, had befriended John many years ago and invited him to holiday meals with his family in Woburn. John had been a drinker for as long as anyone could remember. Three packs of cigarettes a day for over 40 years had likely caused the lung cancer we diagnosed about six months ago. He had come to our Boston City Hospital Clinic to see me about a hacking cough and told me he couldn't eat or sleep and had lost more than 30 pounds. I couldn't hear any breath sounds in his right lung when I examined him, and a chest x-ray showed that the lung was filled with fluid. He didn't seem surprised when I gently told him what we had found, and he acknowledged that for months he had been barely able to breathe when he lay down to sleep at night.

"I was afraid to come see you, Doctor. I didn't want to hear what you are telling me now."

We drained several liters of bloody fluid from his lung, and he called me a hero after he slept soundly for eight hours that night. But the cytology showed malignant cells. Two weeks was about all he could tolerate in the hospital, and he pleaded all the while to go back to the familiar surroundings of Pine Street Inn. He worked on the live-in staff, sorting donations to the clothing room and helping out in the kitchen, and shared a room in the tower with "Machine Gun" Freddy Sullivan, another feisty South Boston Irishman and, like John, a veteran of the Korean War.

The prognosis was grim, a few months at best. After our discussions together with the oncologists, John chose comfort care and no heroic measures. The staff at Pine Street Inn accepted him back for hospice care, something never done before in the shelter. John was able to work several hours a day when he returned, and he came to the Nurses' Clinic for medications each morning and evening. After five good months, he became too feeble to get out of his chair. The live-in staff brought him meals, and the nurses took turns sitting with John through the long night hours. The pleural effusion had begun to accumulate again, and John was increasingly air-hungry but responded to the anti-anxiety medications we gave him. The cancer had spread to his bones and liver, and his intense pain required more frequent doses of morphine. Peggy Thornton, the nurse sitting with John in his room, paged me just before midnight on Friday, May 14, to let me know that he had stopped breathing.

We had finished in the clinic just after 9:30PM that evening. Yoshiko, Marc, and I joined the nurses for our weekly Friday gathering to unwind and share stories. These get-togethers alternated between draughts of Guinness at Doyle's Pub and my home near the Arnold Arboretum where we watched *Miami Vice*, Barbara McInnis' favorite show. Barbara and I drove from Doyle's to the Inn, where I officially pronounced John dead. He had spent a peaceful day, and Peggy said he simply went quietly to sleep. Bill, having already notified the funeral home, drove in from Woburn. Lauretta Woods, the supervisor of the live-in staff who had so staunchly supported John through his ordeal, came immediately from her home in Revere. Donna Scarpa, the clinic's head nurse who had masterfully orchestrated the logistics of end-of-life care in the shelter, rushed over from her home near Worcester Square. I remember sitting with this exhausted and devastated group and marveling at the obscurity in which they accomplished these quiet miracles. Six months earlier John Hennessy had been frightened and alone, fully cognizant of the imminent end of a life he "botched big time." Bill and the remarkable shelter staff offered him the dignity of dying on his own terms, and John died a peaceful and unbroken man.

The Missing International Child

OCTOBER 1988

James Michael Preston created a ruckus outside the clinic at Long Island Shelter one night in the summer of 1988. He was insolent to the nurses, whom he saw as a phalanx trying to divide and conquer his wits. Barbara Blakeney, the nurse practitioner who was the architect of the City of Boston's nursing services for homeless persons and was another of the dynamic and creative women who shaped our service-delivery model, asked me to help negotiate with this vulnerable and frightened man.

"Tell them I don't have bugs!" he shouted above the usual din of the late-evening waiting room at the clinic. I asked him to come into the small area which doubled as an office and an exam room.

"Let me take a look, James, and then I can set them straight and get you to bed."

James was almost 40, with black feline eyes which were at times piercing and at times beguiling, but always sad. His face was creased from too many years wandering in the Florida sun, which was about the only background I knew about James. He told us that he came to Boston when he was arrested in Florida and told to "get out of town or we'll tar and feather you." How he came to Long Island Shelter was a mystery, although that certainly did not set him apart from countless other guests on the Island.

This evening James was agitated and tremulous. He told me that he had been trying to get into bed when one of the counselors asked him to take a shower. Like so many other guests, James riled at the thought. At Pine Street Inn and most of the other adult shelters in town, a shower was required before taking a bed in the dormitory. Many persons chose to come to Long Island because showers were not required unless there was an outbreak of lice or scabies which needed to be controlled. At first I was unsettled by the vehemence, even to the point of giving up a warm bed and leaving the shelter to sleep on the streets, with which some persons rejected showering. But I have come to understand that a shower is a highly complex event for persons whose minds and souls are struggling to protect a tethered reality from relentless voices or frightening delusions.

Showering first of all means parting, albeit temporarily, with one's only possessions. While theft is common in the shelters, the actual fear is that someone will rummage through one's belongings and possess the facts of one's life. Date of birth, true name, driver's license, family pictures, social security number, Medicaid card. To those pursued by the CIA or FBI, parting with such intensely personal information is impossible if one is to survive, and showering in large shelters is intolerable.

James always wore two sets of clothing. He had once explained to me that he kept his wallet and valuables in one pair of trousers and then wore an outer pair just in case anyone tried to pick his pockets. Even in the torrid heat of summer, many homeless persons can be seen on our streets wearing multiple layers of clothing. Our experience has been that often these persons suffer from chronic paranoid schizophrenia and are somehow shielding themselves from the Furies that pursue them—whether voices, visions, parents, lovers, or the CIA. For James, removing the layers of clothing was tantamount to self-revelation and submission to exactly those forces from whom he had spent all his days escaping.

I examined James' scalp and body and thankfully found only an atopic dermatitis. He was no doubt filthy, but he was free of living creatures and entitled to a bed without a shower. In the previous months he had contracted several severe cases of scabies that we had treated in our clinic at the hospital, where we were able to give him a private shower where he could lock the door and keep his belongings with him. Even with such precautions he remained concerned that the room was wired and that the water was contaminated.

"Remember the showers at Auschwitz," he glared.

Through the summer of 1988, James seemed to be decompensating. He kept entirely to himself in the shelter and avoided the nurses and other staff members completely. He would stay out on many nights and would disappear for several weeks at a time. He still came to see me in the shelter clinic on Tuesday and Thursday evenings, but his complaints seemed vague excuses to send signals to "someone who wasn't on their side."

In September he came to our office at the hospital. He was animated and happy, and he wanted me to type his manifesto. As always, he was dressed completely in black, including a knitted woolen hat despite an Indian-summer temperature of 92° in Boston that day.

"This is it. The whole truth."

"What do you mean, James?"

"After all these years of suppression, I've finally been able to remember my past. I have foiled all those attempts to make me forget who I am and where I came from. All their brainwashing techniques were useless, because I'm too smart for them. I am a survivor."

James handed me several pages of handwritten material on a yellow legal pad. He asked me to read it out loud, and he sat back triumphantly in his chair to listen. The rambling fifteen-page tome describes a young boy in the Middle East who survives a massacre in which his parents and siblings are murdered. He is the missing international child sought by the governments of Russia and America, and he must hide on the streets and in the shelters to survive.

"I am condemned. You could never live the way I live because if you ever did you would end up dead. Because you would go out of your mind and end up insane and commit suicide and kill yourself—no money to live on, no home to go to, no family, no friends, no matter where you ever go. You will have to sleep in the streets, along the highways, in the back alley ways, in the open parks, on the benches behind broken-down buildings, in junkyards and in junk cars, in bushes and weeds, and no place to wash, and wearing the same filthy dirty clothes, never washing for days in and days out, and the American people looking at you and laughing at you and giving you very hard looks because you do not have what the American people have. And the American people will not help you one bit at all, even though you never did anything to deserve being treated like this. And if you do ask in a nice way for help, the American people, who have it all, just laugh at you and call you a dirty street bum. Because you cannot make it on your own and there is no way out, because it is so easy to fall into and so very hard to get out of. So you get so low, and then you get to feeling that it's not worth living, so all you think about is death."

James had listened intently through the entire reading, and he cherished a moment of cathartic silence after I finished.

"That is very powerful, James."

"It's just the truth about myself, and the truth is always powerful. You know I could never get this kind of information from any book, and that it has to be the truth."

Clinic was in full swing, and I explained that I wouldn't have time to type the manuscript until the afternoon. He collected the yellow pages, seemed pleased and proud, and left for the MIT library without any explanations.

The following evening at the shelter, James seemed hypomanic. He walked in to see me, but he was very suspicious of the nurses and asked if he could again come to see me in the hospital clinic. He looked bedraggled, his pointed features sharpened by wasted temporal and facial muscles. Both sets of clothing had remained in place since our last meeting, and his hair was now speckled with nits. I couldn't help but notice two large books buried in his jeans and covering his genitalia.

"Protection, James?" I ventured.

"Don't worry about me, I'm a survivor."

James was at the clinic door at Boston City Hospital the following Monday. He had found an attaché case in a downtown dumpster "outside the Hancock Building," and he now had all of his papers stuffed into the case with two belts securing them, just as I once carried my books to grammar school. I had to see one very ill patient before I could see James, and as usual, he frustrated the clinic staff by refusing to wait in the lobby and instead standing in the hallway outside my door. Most people gave him wide berth as they hurried through the morning's business.

Once in the examination room, James took ten minutes to unravel his manuscripts.

"Before we go on," he insisted, "I want to ask you this question, since you are a medical doctor."

"I'll be happy to answer, if I can."

"Why can I never emotionally cry? I never ever shed tears. Even when I saw everything that happened to my parents and my people, I was not able to shed even one tear. I never open up and cry, I only react with anger and frustration. If you went through what I went through, wouldn't you be emotionally upset? Wouldn't you cry?"

I interrupted to answer the question. "I'm sure I would have cried and perhaps I would not have been able to handle such a horrible situation without going insane or at least without seeking someone to counsel me and help me through it." But he wasn't taking my bait.

James sat down and insisted that I read the manifesto again, as there were several new additions. He once again beamed during the reading, and I shuddered at the realization of how little joy or laughter or peace he had been granted in either his real or imagined worlds.

Not much was different, although he had again transcribed the entire manifesto onto yet another yellow pad. I couldn't help but notice the asymmetry of the scattered sections that had been deleted with whiteout and then written over, as if whole periods of our lives can be erased and reconstructed.

The Menagerie

NOVEMBER 1988

Emmylou Davidson paraded into the
office one Wednesday morning in the
fall of 1988. I had known Emmylou
for over three years, through several
hospitalizations for brittle asthma.
She suffered from severe learning
disabilities and chronic schizophrenia,
although several psychiatrists disagreed
on the severity of each. While her
speech was often whiney and childish,
its content was refreshingly unedited,
expletives notwithstanding. Impulse
control was a daily struggle, and
Emmylou was known to have violent
outbursts in the presence of health care
providers and shelter staff.

I had grown very fond of Emmylou, who would often barrage our clinic daily for several weeks and then disappear for months. Usually I would get a forlorn call from an admitting intern in a local emergency room asking for her latest theophylline level, and I would have to humbly explain that such routine care of the asthmatic was nonnegotiable with Emmylou, and blood tests were anathema. Rather, the exact dose of her theophylline was empirically determined by monitoring the wheezes in her lungs during the several-week windows she occasionally granted me. I was quite proud of the ersatz care Emmylou and I had agreed upon, especially since she never returned to physicians who required blood tests. But to beleaguered interns in busy emergency rooms, Emmylou was an unmanageable and inexplicable curse sent by an archaic physician.

Emmylou was 50 years old but dressed and acted as a young child. Her trademark pigtails had an array of brightly colored animal-shaped barrettes. She always wore either Mickey Mouse ears or a beanie similar to the ones worn by Spanky and the Rascals. Her clothes were all bright yellow and pink, and her blouses usually had repetitive animal designs. Emmylou was barely five feet tall and markedly overweight, and her Mary Jane shoes dangled freely when she sat in the examination room chair. Her eyes were gigantic through thick Coke-bottle glasses, and her prominent overbite and shiny white teeth divided a sea of cheeks, completing the childish aura. Garfield was her bosom buddy, and most of Boston had encountered the unforgettable pair on the MBTA. Today, however, Emmylou had a stroller in which she had Garfield and three new stuffed animals. All had been dressed in appropriate children's clothing which had been acquired last week at a sale in Filene's basement, and Emmylou spent several minutes tending to "the kids" after she brought the entourage into my office. Garfield took his customary place on top of my typewriter, while two balding monkeys were put on the floor to frolic.

"I'm going to Disneyland from November third until the seventh, so I want to schedule the operation on November eighth."

Emmylou's small incisional hernia was of great concern to her.

Several times she had presented to the shelter clinic with abdominal pain and vomiting and pleaded for relief from these "hernia attacks." While her hernia was small and needed an elective repair, it was not likely the cause of these symptoms that surfaced in times of great anxiety or when she wanted to be given medical authorization to remain inside a shelter during the day hours. We had arranged the surgery twice previously, and both times she had elected to forego the procedure as she was wheeled into the operating theater. I dreaded the thought of trying to convince the surgeons to try again, given how valuable operating room time is.

"Emmylou, we will have to think of ways to help with your anxiety if we try to schedule the surgery again. Are you still living at Parker Street?"

Parker Street Shelter is located at the Erich Lindemann Mental Health Center, one of three transitional shelters for the chronic mentally ill. Emmylou had been "pink-papered" several weeks ago and committed to a psychiatric facility for bizarre and threatening behavior. Her discharge plan had included time at Parker Street with careful supervision of her medications.

"The place sucks. I'm allergic to the fucking cigarettes. And the place is all walls. There's one window, but as far as I'm concerned it's just a glass wall. It doesn't even open, so how can it be a window? It's a wall. Amen."

She stopped to rearrange the stuffed animals, took Garfield onto her lap, and told me she was spending this week at Rosie's Place, her favorite shelter. Rosie's is a beautiful facility just around the corner from the hospital with twenty beds for women. Roses are put at each woman's dinner place, and the guests are served dinner by volunteers—small reminders of the dignity and respect each woman deserves but rarely experiences during life on the streets. Because of demand on the beds, each woman is given seven nights at Rosie's, after which she must wait one month before returning. Rosie's is a marked contrast to the harsher realities of Parker Street Shelter.

"How many more nights do you have at Rosie's?"

"Only two more."

"Will you then return to Parker Street?"

"Oh God! I call that place a torture chamber. I'm not a well person. You can't just take someone with hernias and asthma as bad as mine and stick them outdoors and then scream later that she's sick. I want out of that place any way I can.

"I just wanted to tell you about the horrible things that have been happening to me. It's like living in a nightmare. I'm so fucking afraid of being evaluated, sent over to the Mass General, strapped to a bed for nothing, whether you're good or bad for their psych evaluation you automatically get handcuffed to the bed, one foot and one leg, by the hour, and sometimes overnight. I'm so afraid of that, Doctor, that I hear ambulances when there aren't any there. You're an M.D., and you know god-dammed well that isn't a good sign. They love to keep me so fucking afraid, and I just get so nervous and frightened."

Tears poured forth at this point, but she insisted on talking through them.

"I tell you what it's equal to. Take a look at your Vietnam kids, take a look at your Central American babies. You ask them what it's like to live through a war and they just keep quiet until they draw you a picture of a man with his head blown off. Now you tell me if that's good!"

Emmylou had been audibly wheezing throughout her diatribe, and I was relieved to finally get to the medical issue at hand. The health care of homeless women is an art I have been learning from the nurses in the clinics at Pine Street Inn, Long Island Shelter, the Women's Lunch Place, and Rosie's Place. The prevalence of severe and persistent mental illness among single adult women is high, and our experience has suggested that most unattached homeless women living chronically in the shelters and on the streets have suffered untold physical, sexual, and emotional trauma. Schizophrenia and bipolar disorder, as well as affective and personality disorders, are common. Substance use among homeless women is relatively rare and usually an attempt to cope with an underlying psychiatric disorder. The journey toward homelessness is sinuous and treacherous for women, and I can only guess at the horrors and torment these women have experienced.

Emmylou, like many homeless women, would never have allowed me to examine her until she felt comfortable in my presence. I have had to learn the difficult lesson of vigilant patience, something the frenetic pace of my profession does not understand. Emmylou would have walked out of the exam room had I shown any impatience or tried to hurry her along.

This morning she was audibly wheezing and had a hacking cough productive of thick, white sputum. Her lungs were otherwise unremarkable on exam, and her heart rhythm was slow and regular. She had stopped taking her theophylline because she was jittery and sleepless at night. We compromised. She promised to use her steroid inhaler, and we prescribed a once-a-day preparation of theophylline that she would try each morning. No blood tests were even suggested.

Finally, Emmylou carted her small menagerie out of the office with an agreement to return in one week and a promise to go back to Parker Street until her asthma was better. I called to be sure she would be allowed to remain inside for a few days until she recovered. I smiled. We both had gotten what we wanted.

Emmylou returned to clinic one week later with her asthma in good control. Once again she wheeled in the animals, all with new outfits obtained at a bazaar at the Church of the Covenant.

"The women at the shelter are giving me more static. Now we have problems with sex, and I wish you would do something about it. The other night I was speaking about sex, gay sex. I'm gay, but you know that. What's wrong with that? And then this holy-roller supervisor came and told us to stop talking. I said one swear word, fuck, and she told me that if I swore again I would be put outside for an hour. Christianity sucks. I left right away and spent the night at Day is Done, just to get them worried."

Day is Done is a small storefront near Fenway Park with twelve couches and a couple of easy chairs where women can spend the night. The mostly volunteer staff members serve a small number of homeless women in an alternative setting to the larger, more impersonal shelters. While only open nights from 8PM until 7AM, Day is Done offers a welcome refuge for women seeking the intimacy of a small community.

"I don't have much that I can fight back with, but if I do my bit to disappear for a few nights and not report in, then maybe they'll bar me and I will be free of them at last. What they've done to me is abuse, it goes under the heading of abuse to women and abuse to people in shelters. I won't stand for it, but I don't have any power to stop them."

She cried for about a minute and stopped abruptly.

"Hey, how do you like his outfit?" She held up Garfield, who was dressed in a yellow summer dress.

"Very nice, Emmylou, where did you find it?"

"Jordan Marsh. I got the dress for two dollars, pretty good, huh? I also got this shirt, and if you look carefully there's elephants, tigers, kangaroos, giraffes, and even a rhinoceros."

Emmylou also had on several unusual bracelets that appeared to be square pieces of porcelain, brightly colored, with round holes for the wrist in the middle. I told Emmylou that I liked them and found them most unusual.

"You'll die when you hear this. I took the new theophylline the other morning and the pill got caught in my throat. Everybody thought I was choking or something. So they called the ambulance and took me to Mass General. I wouldn't go without the kids, so they let me take the stroller."

"That must have raised a few eyebrows, Emmylou."

"Everybody was afraid to ask me about the kids, but I didn't give a shit. When they decided I wasn't choking to death, they sent me over to the Walk-in Clinic to see if maybe it was an allergy to the medicine or something. So they put me in a wheelchair and the nurse pushed me while I pushed the kids. Fuck 'em if they can't take a joke."

Wonderland

FEBRUARY 1989

Jeremiah Noonan showed me his checkbook to prove his point. He had depleted his life savings of almost ten thousand dollars as a guest of the Copley Square Hotel for the past six months, and this was his second night at Long Island Shelter. Tentative and guarded, this elderly man unfolded his story slowly.

A veteran of World War II, Mr. Noonan was now 75. After the war he had been a laborer in a potato shed for a dozen years, "Making peanuts to go with my potato chips." He was hired by Harvard College as a maintenance worker and compiled an impeccable record for eleven years. From then until his retirement in 1980, he worked the graveyard shift cleaning toilets at Jordan Marsh Department Store on Washington Street. For almost 30 years he lived in a rooming house on Broadway in Everett.

"Nothing fancy, just four walls, a bureau, a cot, and a bathroom down the hall. Didn't need much else."

He didn't smoke or drink, and he never married. He never bothered to get a radio or a television, and he had no phone. Wonderland Racetrack was his passion, and he rode the MBTA each evening to enjoy the atmosphere and to bet on his favorite greyhounds before heading to work. The rent had gone from eight to twenty dollars per week during three decades, but urban redevelopment finally lured the aging owners to sell, and this septuagenarian was homeless for the first time in his life. Elder Services somehow found him a foster home in Revere. After four years he absconded under a cloud of innuendo and paranoia that he refuses to discuss. He decided to stay at the Copley Square Hotel until his savings were completely drained. He had been on the streets for several weeks before finally seeking refuge here at Long Island Shelter.

"I'm glad to have the chance to speak with a medical doctor. I must be discreet, and I've been nervous about all these psychiatric nurses and social workers hanging around me. These last years have been very trying."

The door to the exam room was ajar, and he reached over to close it.

"Troubles and loneliness have been faithful companions all my life. They wouldn't even let me fight in the war, they just threw me in a hospital and fried, poached, and scrambled my brain. When they finally let me out, I was one horny hunk without a thought to call my own. I tried to kiss a girl on Monument Hill in Charlestown and she threw the book at me. Since I couldn't read, and the judge was so disgusted, I got tossed into Westborough State Hospital and they buzzed my goddamned noggin again. Should have shaved my horns, though, because I was out in eight months and women still seemed irresistible. Work helped keep me exhausted, but one weekend in the Public Gardens I saw two beautiful girls walking together and I pranced up and kissed one of them right smack on the lips. She got angry just like the other one, and I was off to Westborough State for the next two years. Told me if I tried anything like that again, they'd have to operate on one of my lobes."

Jeremiah managed to stay out of trouble after that, although it wasn't clear just how. Work and the track seemed his only activities, other than Sunday masses. As I pieced the scenario together, he had been marginally able to cope until he lost his room in Everett. During these past four years with his foster family in Revere, he decompensated and was now in flight.

"They've been trailing me all my life, and now that I've run away they're hunting me like an animal and torturing me with this VCR machine. Sure, everything seemed fine at first, and they told me I'd be part of the family. Used to eat dinner with the widow and her two sons, and then she and I would sit in the parlor and watch TV the whole evening. Two years ago this special machine with blue flickering lights shows up under the TV, and she tells me it belongs to Tommy so he can make home movies. But I recognized that discontinued military machine used in the war to transmit mental conversations and deliver painful heat waves."

"That's when the aches and pains in my shoulders and hips began. I would be lying in bed at night, and I could hear that machine and a lot of laughing, and pretty soon they'd zap me and I'd scream in pain. And each time I tried to fall asleep, another series of zaps. By Christmas time, three of those VCRs were in the house—one in the parlor, and one in Joe's room, and one in Tommy's. They started to manipulate me by using double and triple-strength heat waves, and they even found they could make me impotent. Every time I got a hard-on, zap, zap. When the police joined the laughter, I knew I had to make a run for it, so I dismantled two of the three machines, took my bankbook, and hid out at the Copley Place Hotel."

"Soon they fixed the VCRs and zeroed in on my thoughts and whereabouts. They wouldn't let me sleep longer than two hours at a time without heat waves to my toes, knees, and hips. When I slept on the bed, the waves could come directly through the window. I found that I could block many of them by sleeping on the floor behind the drapes, and so I spent three months on the floor. They can send their thoughts directly to me, and they've made it very clear how angry they are about my leaving Revere without saying good-by to their mother.

"'We will annihilate you, but we don't want to kill you now. You stayed here four years, and we'll torture you for four years and then kill you.'"

Mr. Noonan stopped and stood up abruptly.

"They're listening now, I've got to go."

Several calls to local agencies and the Department of Mental Health failed to uncover any information about Mr. Noonan. While this elderly gentleman's paranoia was nothing short of hell-on-earth, he sadly did not meet any of the criteria for mandatory treatment. My suggestion of a small dose of Haldol to help with sleep met with a stolid rejection a week later when he returned to see me in the shelter clinic.

From a medical perspective, Mr. Noonan had severe osteoarthritis of his hips and knees, which probably accounted for the sharp zapping pains. Well-developed cataracts of both eyes had caused considerable deterioration in vision over the past several years, although he had chosen to avoid the eye doctors.

"They've been working on my eyes for some time, I know that. Acetic acid and arsenic are vaporized by the VCRs and transmitted through the air, up my nostrils, and into the eyes. I finally went to see the doctor this week, and he told me that an operation could fix the problem. So I've been trying to appease Tommy and Joe, because I know that they could just destroy my eyes after the operation, or worse, they might be crazy enough to cripple the doctor's fingers during the surgery and leave me blind!"

I offered assurances of protection and even suggested that some of the medicines might well block the heat waves, but Mr. Noonan was inconsolable. His tie was askew, and I couldn't help but notice the dried egg yolk on his buttondown collar. His thick, calloused hands were tanned and wrinkled, and his nose blue and bulbous. Tufts of thick white hair seemed planted in his ears. I felt entirely helpless, humiliated that I could not reach out to this aged, tormented soul. However crazy and far-fetched so much of this was to me, to Mr. Noonan all was vividly real, and he was living in the depths of hell.

"I spoke to Elise the psych nurse last night. She was very clever and got a lot out of me. And today they've been giving me hell. Arms, chest, legs, back. And my eyes burn. And they've been zapping my penis constantly. When Elise asked me if I've ever heard any voices, I had to honestly tell her no. I know what she's driving at, and she means mental voices. I told her no, because I hear real voices."

Odd Angles

JANUARY 1990

I have learned never to judge. Things are
seldom what they seem on the streets
or in the shelters. The hearts and souls
covered by ulcers and infestations and
shielded by the patois of Dorchester and
South Boston are unpredictable and
almost always hidden. Medicine has
always been intertwined with religion,
and I recall reading about the fervent
search for the anatomical location of the
soul by physicians in the Middle Ages.

While the heart seemed most likely, many opted for the brain. A staunch group thought that the liver, that whirring metabolic factory in the abdomen, was the hidden reservoir of the soul.

Adam Innisfree had been coming intermittently to the clinic for four years, usually after taking a "header" during an alcoholic blackout or during a seizure. Those with long years of drinking alcohol often walk with a wide-based gait to counter the disequilibrium caused by alcohol's effects on the cerebellum in the brain. During a fall, the legs are rigid, and the feet become the fulcrum of the fall. The sound of the skull slamming into the concrete sidewalk or tile floors from six feet up is nauseating, and the head invariably bounces up and slams back down a second and third time. I cringed at first hearing this sound when a man fell during a blackout at Pine Street Inn, and only then did I understand the extent of the damage to the brain tissue sustained by those with repeated falls over the years.

Usually very private, Adam burst into the clinic quite agitated last September, and it was to be the last time I would see him. Adam was learned, articulate, and provocative, an observant chronicler of wasted lives and falls from grace. His imposing 6-foot-5-inch frame underscored his patrician mannerisms, although this evening his armor was dented by a blackened right eye and a jagged laceration of the forehead.

"I came to see Betsy, sweet Betsy from Pike, I call her."

Betsy Kendrick had been a nurse at the Pine Street Inn Clinic since the early 1980's. She was a dynamo of energy with a knack for reaching those most frightened by systems and shelters. She had recently attempted to stop smoking, a cause for much skepticism and a few lotteries among the clinic staff. I asked Adam how Betsy was doing with her smoking cessation program.

"I've frankly never seen her smoke. Nicotine, they say, is the perfect drug. It's both a depressant and a stimulant at the same time. Menthol is another kick. If I stop smoking menthols for a while, and I suddenly buy a package of Kools, which are very strong anyway, I feel excellent! Back in the 60's when I smoked grass—I no longer do—we used to lay off menthols for about six weeks, and then a single menthol cigarette would give us a kick. Just the menthol!

"Yet it was very mild, especially when compared to smoking grass or dropping acid. Did you know that acid is a derivative of a wheat rust? True, it's synthesized now, but in medieval villages in Western Europe the wheat crop would be afflicted with this rust, a type of fungus actually, which was not destroyed during the baking process. The bread was eaten, and whole villages became mad."

Adam was a fountain of such information, and I cherished his visits. A perplexing rash of his lower extremities had erupted last week, and we sent a picture to Dr. Ernesto Gonzalez, our guardian angel in the Dermatology Department at Massachusetts General Hospital, who quickly diagnosed nummular psoriasis. We had given Adam the recommended steroid cream, and his legs improved dramatically. Alcohol was always a sensitive subject to broach. I was surprised at Adam's chuckle when I asked how he was managing what he always called "the battle of the bottle." He retorted with his characteristic and worn-out refrain.

"I'd rather have a bottle in front of me than a frontal lobotomy. I know you're sick of that. But to tell the truth, I've recently been detoxified at Central Hospital in Somerville. It's like a country club, and I highly recommend it to anyone who has Medicaid. This was the first detox I have ever been in."

I was surprised and overjoyed. For four years I had tried to convince Adam to take a break from his daily bottle or two of vodka, but he disdained detoxes and groups and 12-step programs.

"I loathe getting in touch with my feelings. All that crap about my inner child and my codependency—hell, what feelings? I'm a good old-fashioned drunk!"

Some years ago he recalled suffering "a very small and a very trivial heart attack." His electrocardiogram showed evidence of an old infarction in the inferior aspect of his heart, but I was never able to convince Adam to give us permission to send for the hospital records in another state. He had no interest in letting me schedule an exercise tolerance test, and he didn't feel he needed the aspirin and beta blocker that I recommended for medication. He often rushed into the clinic frightened by chest pains, but he refused to let us send him to the emergency room. He chose rather to treat his chest pain with rest and alcohol and "not necessarily in that order."

"Betsy and I have a little joke between us. With this terrible chronic infection on my ankle, I keep asking Betsy for a McBandage each day. She has a blackboard behind the door with two golden arches:

Nurses' Clinic, Over 5 Billion Served. This Week's Special: McEnema!

"My tuberculous skin test was positive last year, making me a converter. Barbara McInnis suggested isoniazid for nine months, since my chest x-ray was entirely clear. She also suggested another drug that begins with an R."

I explained that the additional medication we have been recommending is rifampin. Over 60 cases of active pulmonary tuberculosis had been diagnosed among homeless adults living at Pine Street Inn in the mid-1980s, with almost half resistant to two commonly used antibiotics, isoniazid and streptomycin. While none of the persons with active tuberculosis had AIDS, people who were immuno-compromised were at greater risk for developing active disease, and I sensed the desperation behind Adam's rare willingness to consider detoxification and to discuss personal concerns about his physical health. He looked embarrassed and ashamed.

"And I would ask a favor, if you don't mind. I would like to have an HIV test. A close friend of mine and I broke up after he refused to consider taking the test. The only thing I could possibly do was cut that relationship dead and get an HIV test. It seems like a good idea, especially if I can pick up that tuberculosis germ so easily in the shelter."

"Have you had an HIV test done before?"

"Oh yes, Cambridge Hospital and Brigham and Women's. I just consider it responsible behavior. You need both the ELISA test and the Western Blot. I'm fairly certain it will come out negative.

"I plan to write two books in the near future. One is almost a necessity, the other just an indulgence. The first is a memoir entitled

Boston on Zero Dollars a Day: Homeless in the Hub. I hope to do for homelessness what Jonathan Kozol did for education with *Death at an Early Age*. He precipitated the entire Boston school crisis and won a Pulitzer Prize as well!

"About two years ago I broke my leg on one of Mayor Flynn's cracked sidewalks. I had a long leg cast and had to sleep for two months on a cot in the lobby because I couldn't go upstairs safely. That was the first and only bone I have ever broken. I've been lucky at the age of 47 ...my birthday was one week ago.

"When I awakened one morning, the young fellow next to me was dead. He had been dumped on the mat by the cops and the EMTs in the middle of the night. Paul was his name, just 22 years old and he died of internal bleeding. Apparently he had liver problems.

"I will memorialize Paul in my book. Father Amory knows his name and I will find out more about him. I don't see enough of Father Amory these days, as he spends much of his time at Haley House, the Catholic Worker place. Did you know that he spent fifteen years in the Philippines as a missionary? He lives in Cambridge now, at the residence for the LaSalette Fathers between Harvard and Porter Squares. He has worked with Mitch Snyder in Washington at CCNV. Now he has quite a ministry at Pine Street Inn, and he has told his superior where to get off. He quit drinking but always has a cigarette in his mouth, so he understands the guests in the shelter very well and speaks their language. He still says his Breviary every night. He's a fascinating man. He's wearing the dog collar recently, so he must be getting conservative in his old age! He has always worn the pectoral cross, which is a lovely thing. I had one, smaller than that, in ebony, and blessed by the Pope, for God's sake. Someone gave it to me, and I wore it until the figure dropped off. You have to think about the symbolism of that...perhaps I have dropped off the cross finally, the cross of my own demise. I have been party to my own destruction.

"But Paul died, and the EMTs came in, and it was 3:20 in the morning. Tragic. But I'm used to tragedy. The man sleeping in the bed next to me died in his sleep, drove me crazy. I never met the guy other than in his final repose. I went to public schools, but my mother tells me that I was correcting her grammar by the time I was three. It runs in the family. And I attended the Chicago Institute of Music, and I sang with the Philadelphia Orchestra. At the age of 8, I had my own radio show that lasted about two years. I hosted my own television show later. I was a volunteer astronomer for the Cambridge Observatory. And the Massachusetts Rehabilitation Commission wants me to go to Bunker Hill Community College and become a bookkeeper. See what I mean? It does not make sense at all.

"The other book I'm contemplating is a coffee table book. I've also been a professional photographer. Mostly industrial. Commonwealth Avenue happens to be one of the great boulevards of the world, one of the masterpieces of urban planning. I would like to do a book of close-ups, not only of monuments, but also of the architectural details of those magnificent buildings along Commonwealth Avenue as far as Massachusetts Avenue. I would definitely need a bellows camera. The focal plane needs to be frequently changed, and the lens can be tilted in a variety of ways with a bellows camera. One can correct odd angles this way. This book is an indulgence for my own pleasure, a form of mental masturbation. The first book is demanding to be written soon."

Adam seemed troubled and reflective. He asked me to renew his blood pressure medication, and he wandered off into the South End. Two mornings later the Medical Examiner called to let me know Adam was found bludgeoned to death in a parking lot a block from the shelter. He was unrecognizable and identified only by his fingerprints.

The Bear

JULY 1992

Just after midnight on July 4th of 1992, the van workers and I came upon the makeshift memorial near Jack Anderson's park bench in Commonwealth Park near Kenmore Square. A rose had been tacked to a nearby tree, along with a picture of Jack above an arresting image of a fully upright grizzly bear. A card was inscribed by street friends and neighbors. It included notes from the children who play most days in the park. We had known and cared for Jack for years on the streets of Boston, but we had never seen the playful soul who so loved children.

Jack Anderson, or "Bear" to all of us, had been found dead next to his bench a few days earlier. He and Indian Jimmy had suffered head trauma and rib fractures when a car hit them near Fenway Park in early June, and both had been sent from the hospital to recuperate at McInnis House. A week before his death Bear absconded and found his way back to his makeshift home in his park. When we brought him soup and sandwiches late the next night, he politely resisted all entreaties and bribes to return to Barbara McInnis House, and he staunchly refused to go to the shelter. The whiskey had restored his familiar boisterous laugh and gruff demeanor, and he proudly growled that he was "back in the lair where I belong."

Jack had wandered Kenmore Square and Back Bay with a pack of insouciant post-modern exiles, characters worthy of Bret Harte's campfires, scornful of traditional society and barely surviving at its cruel and bitter fringes. Pine Street Inn's outreach van has been a literal lifeline of soup and sandwiches and blankets to these fiercely independent individuals who sleep in the streets and parks, on fire escapes and grates, under bridges and highways, and near the river-banks of Boston. Wandering the urban desert as prophets unfettered by material possessions and shunned by their own families and people, they view their ostracism with biblical nobility and angrily acknowl-edge this banishment to the fringes of a wanton society. Many street names echo this theme: Simon the Elder, Isaiah with AIDS, Matthew Zion, Ezekiel from Cuba. The eccentricities are spellbinding, much like "the subterranean twilit characters of the metropolis" in Joseph Mitchell's *Up in the Old Hotel*. No doubt Mitchell's Joe Gould, the drinker struggling to complete his translation of Longfellow's poetry into the language of seagulls while awaiting the publication of his magnum opus, *An Oral History of Our Time*, would have been com-fortable hanging out with Bear.

I'm not sure how or when Jack Anderson came to be called Bear; some thought it went back to his days in the Marine Corps, others suspected a self-chosen sobriquet to protect the mystery that envel-oped his life. Whatever the origin, the ursine myth was embellished with characteristic aplomb. A thick red-brown beard matched his burly and foreboding presence, while he often boasted of "hibernating" on the Boston University grates during the coldest winters and subsisting on the spoils of dumpster diving along the Back Bay alleys. A no-holds-barred street brawler, Bear had innumerable visits to the emergency departments of Massachusetts General Hospital and the old Boston City Hospital for stab wounds and head trauma. He alternately charmed and exasperated his caregivers with his laughter and cockiness. Bear always claimed that he was born in Scandinavia and some "good and loving folks" had adopted and raised him near Old Saybrook, Connecticut. He spoke of a stint in a state hospital when he was seventeen "for violent tendencies." Drinking and disorderly conduct resulted in a dishonorable discharge from his beloved Marine Corps, and he survived by working as a bouncer, construction laborer, and security officer. Jack Anderson was not his given name but rather his proud and not-too-subtle American version of Hans Christian Andersen. His life was legendary on the streets but hardly a fairy tale. We never found his given name, and Bear's body lay unclaimed in the city morgue for six months before he was laid to rest in the paupers' cemetery alongside countless other homeless men and women who have died on Boston's streets.

Frostbitten

FEBRUARY 2000

On the first Monday of this century, we basked in 60-degree moonlight on Pine Street Inn's outreach van. The following week winter appeared in sudden and stark relief with temperatures plunging into the single digits and wind-chill factors of 30–40 degrees below zero. We all knew it was coming, but the luxurious lull of an unseasonably warm December had us looking past the winter with delusions of spring.

The dramatic change in temperature was felt throughout the homeless community. While the outreach teams coaxed many of the most independent street dwellers into shelter, about 50 persons found places to sleep on the streets and under the bridges.

The most dangerous times for exposure injuries to the cold can be the shoulder seasons of winter, when warm days are followed by cold nights. People fall asleep in the relative warm and are not adequately protected to withstand the nighttime cold. Our worst case of hypothermia occurred in 1989 in October, when the temperature was a balmy 45 degrees during the day but fell to 22 degrees that night. A chronic rough sleeper and self-proclaimed survivalist was drinking in the early evening and, covered by a single blanket, fell asleep in a doorway. His body temperature was 64 degrees when he was found in the morning. He survived but was left with severe cognitive and neurological impairments, and he has been in a nursing home since that time.

The precipitous plunge in temperature occurred on the night of January 16. Stephen Tremble was found prone on the sidewalk in the Financial District at 7AM and was rushed to Massachusetts General Hospital with a core body temperature of 72 degrees. Within an hour of his arrival in the emergency department, EMS were called to a dumpster next to the Boston Garden, home of the Celtics and the Bruins and about two blocks from the hospital. Joe Carter had fallen asleep in his usual dumpster and was rushed to the emergency room with a core body temperature of 70 degrees. Both men were unknown and without identification upon arrival at the hospital. In a heroic effort to warm them, doctors rushed them to the operating room and placed them on cardio-pulmonary by-pass, a procedure used primarily during open-heart surgery to divert blood from the heart and provide oxygen. Both "unknown males" then went to the Surgical Intensive Care Unit for continued warming. Dr. Cary W. Akins, the extraordinary and legendary cardiac surgeon at Massachusetts General Hospital, called and asked if we could help identify the two men. Both men were well known to us, and we were able to work closely

with the specialists in caring for them. Both survived without notice-
able cognitive impairment, a tribute to the efforts and rapid response
of the surgeons at Massachusetts General Hospital. After a week, Joe
and Stephen were transferred to our McInnis House for continued
care. Interestingly, both sustained only mild frostbite to the toes despite the profound hypothermia. Both recounted vivid memories of
their near-death experiences, each noting a period of euphoria and
calm that followed the initial shivering in the painful cold. Survivors
of hypothermia often describe a sense of "floating in the air" and experience an intense warmth that can lead them to shed their clothes,
a circumstance known as "paradoxical undressing."

Several other individuals sustained varying degrees of frostbite
during January. Six of these were admitted to McInnis House with
severe frostbite of the feet or hands. Another two individuals remain
in Boston Medical Center with infections and other complications of
frostbite. One Albanian-speaking gentleman who was found freezing
in the back of a van near Carson Beach in South Boston will likely
lose both feet.

An elderly and hard-working homeless man from the Caribbean
is in McInnis House with blackened feet sustained when he was earning money shoveling snow. His diabetes is complicated by a dense
peripheral neuropathy that has left him with little sensation of pain
or position in his feet. He continued working because he felt no pain,
and when he took off his boots in the shelter he was horrified to see
the damage to his feet. One foot has become necrotic from the toes to
halfway along the foot. This area will soon fall off, and he will require
an operation to cover the exposed area with skin grafts.

Frostbite is perhaps the most emblematic complication of homelessness. It occurs within minutes to hours to people whose lives and
limbs have been numbed, blackened, and broken by the complexities
and vicissitudes of a life spent in persistent poverty. One gentleman
who has lived on the streets for years, pursued by his own Furies, calls
himself an urban nomad, "exiled from the warm glow inside those
brownstones on Commonwealth Avenue." He has endured three epi-

sodes of frostbite, resulting in the loss of several fingers as well as the permanent loss of feeling in one foot.

"My circulation has been cut off. I just can't feel anything anymore."

Another young Puerto Rican gentleman with schizophrenia and alcoholism spent almost a year at McInnis House in 1994 with frostbite of all ten toes. He anguished along with our staff as the tissue demarcated over several months, and many toes fell off, to his horror and that of his caregivers. During this current cold spell six years later, he sustained frostbite of fingers in both hands and will undergo more disfigurement and disability as he loses bits of these fingers over the next months.

Frostbite is a physical and psychic drama played in slow motion and underscored by constant pain and the horror of watching fingers and toes become necrotic, blacken, and eventually fall off (called "auto-amputation" in the medical world). Entirely preventable, the suffering and disfigurement from frostbite are indelible, and the costs incalculable.

These patient portraits on the following pages were taken by Dr. O'Connell. ▶

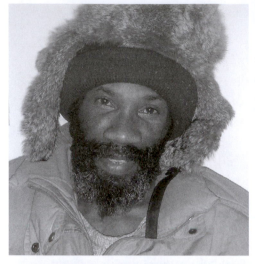
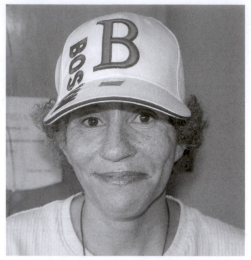
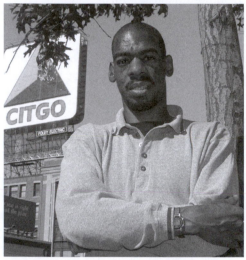
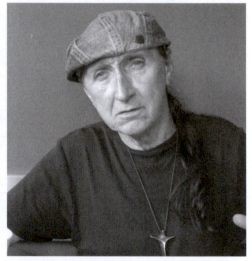
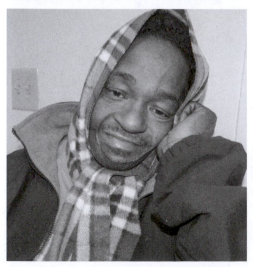
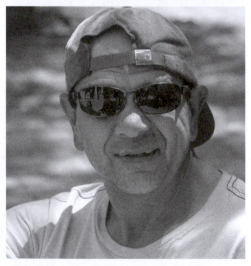

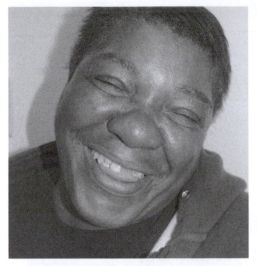 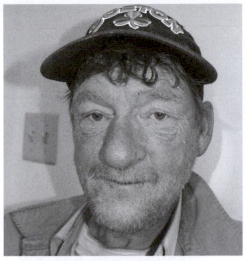

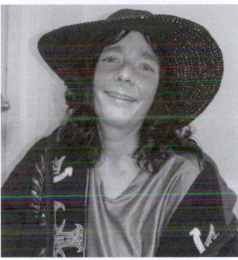 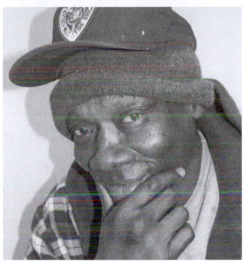

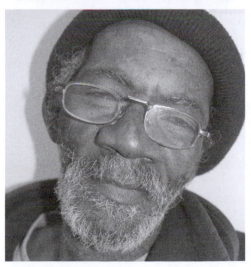 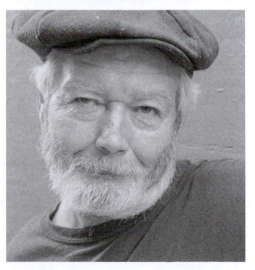

Blessings that Sustain

OCTOBER 2000

The devastation from Annemarie's death permeated our street team for weeks, and the reverberations linger still. Despite death's starkly familiar presence on the streets and our steely clinical grit from years of caring for those exposed to the extremes of weather, Annemarie—young, bright, charismatic, and full of promise— had gotten under our skin. As her doctor through many turbulent years, I had become fond of this proud, exacting, and often insolent 38-year-old woman.

With pert smile and imperial stubbornness, Annemarie had, on the afternoon before her death, departed New England Medical Center's emergency department as soon as the x-rays had failed to find fractures beneath her bruised and swollen face. A week earlier she had histrionically hailed Pine Street Inn's outreach van from her bench on Boston Common around midnight. Bristling through shakes and tremors, she demanded a bed and posthaste transportation to her favorite detox on Boston's Long Island.

I knew to brace myself in the wake of any formal salutation.

"Doctor O'Connell, you're in charge of the detox and I'm sick. Call now and arrange a bed. Be sure that Janet is the nurse on duty tonight. I had a drink about fifteen minutes ago, and I'll need Librium in less than an hour."

Such captivating and infuriating entitlement—urine-stained jeans and muddied sweatshirt notwithstanding—belied a fraying dignity and spiraling despair. Despite the late hour, the nurses were happy to make a bed available, and Annemarie's irrepressible charm lightened the ride down the expressway. We could not help but succumb to her laughter and heavily cloaked gratitude. All compliments were barbed.

"Why the hell do you work on the van, Doc? You should be home sleeping. I need you to be awake tomorrow so that you can figure out why I'm having these pains in my stomach! But no mind, Denny will figure it out faster than you anyway."

As she had promised during the ride to Long Island, Annemarie completed five days of medical detoxification from alcohol, but she decided to forego the 28-day program that had been so helpful to her in the past. She left for the streets two days before her death.

We aren't sure how she sustained the facial trauma that led to her emergency room visit, but afterward she met an old friend and slept under her usual tree on Boston Common. She mentioned that she was tired and wanted to join her late boyfriend, Sam. Pine Street Inn's outreach van staff saw her sleeping comfortably under blankets around 3AM. She never awakened. At the outdoor memorial service led by Reverend Deborah Little of the Cathedral on the Common, Annemarie's brother shared tender memories framed by family pictures of a bright and mischievous toddler and a proud and strikingly beautiful high school graduate. Her ashes were placed in Sam's grave.

We had rooted for her to beat the odds. Hours of care and concern would surely help quiet the Furies that relentlessly pursued her clear across childhood to her deathbed on the Common. She had borne more sadness, been offered fewer choices, and suffered through more physical and sexual violence than any of us could imagine. Death dashed all hope of success and opened Pandora's box anew for us: do our efforts make a difference, or is this litany of suffering and death inexorable?

Caring for homeless people has been my full-time job for more than fifteen years. I suspect that the joy I find in my job bespeaks a deep character flaw, a subject I puzzle over often with my close friend and hero, Pedro Jose Greer. A Cuban-American physician who has worked miracles in caring for homeless people and refugees in Miami for years, he is rapier quick and paraphrases Yeats, who noted that the Irish are a people whose sense of impending tragedy and guilt has remained constant throughout the centuries despite brief moments of unmitigated joy. While this essay could no doubt plumb the tragedy, I would prefer to seize the joy.

A number of unanticipated blessings have protected me through the years. First, medicine still fascinates me. The acuity, complexity, and breadth of illness among homeless persons is bewildering, from AIDS and tuberculosis through exposures to the weather, infestations, and the management of chronic diseases. For those who love the science of medicine, the burden of disease is compelling, the need great, and the clinical challenges truly exhilarating.

Second, the long art needed to implement the science has an equal allure: how do we reach out to bring the best of medicine to those who are living in persistent poverty on the margins of our society?

The nursing profession, so often our muse in medicine, imparts a third blessing with a simple observation. Health care for the disenfranchised is predicated upon a one-to-one relationship made possible only by the investment of time and by a willingness to venture beyond offices and exam rooms to unfamiliar turf. Caring for homeless persons requires us to engage in many of the very human activities that originally enticed me to become a doctor: to listen to stories, to be available, to share in sorrows and joys, to ease suffering, to make an occasional difference. The layered paradox of an urban service-delivery model that harkens back to the days of the country doctor is difficult to escape: care is best brought to homeless people and families by "home" visits in the shelters and on the streets.

A fourth blessing comes with learning to do no harm. A paralyzing sense of anger and discouragement is commonplace for our BHCHP doctors during the first year on the job. Despite efforts aimed at finding safe and affordable housing, the cycle of homelessness can seem intractable, our efforts hopeless, and our advocacy futile.

The final blessing is an embarrassment of riches for which I am deeply grateful. During residency, I noticed that those caring for excluded populations risked becoming marginalized within the medical profession. Several guardian angels assuaged my fears and assured me that this would not happen. From the first day I arrived at Harvard Medical School, our Dean of Students, Dr. Daniel Federman, encouraged me to learn well but follow the heart. Throughout these three decades, he has been a steadfast and wise mentor, always finding ways within the medical school's curriculum to celebrate the care of poor and vulnerable populations. At Massachusetts General Hospital, Drs. John Potts, George Thibeault, and the irrepressible Thomas Durant created a professional career path for me within an academic teaching hospital that has remained my home base. Dr. John Noble of Boston City Hospital, Dr. Sandy Lamb of Boston's Department of Health and Hospitals, and Dr. Joseph Cohen of the Lemuel Shattuck Hospital forged our program's model and overcame innumerable obstacles to help BHCHP succeed. The importance of the collegiality and encouragement of many remarkable physicians, teachers, and friends cannot be overstated, and I offer heartfelt thanks. Indeed, how could any life succumb to ennui surrounded by such munificence?

Imponderables

AUGUST 2001

One of our most endearing rough sleepers died last Tuesday at Boston Medical Center, one week past his 36th birthday. Raised by nuns in an orphanage in Pawtucket, Brian Depeche cloaked much of his past in mystery and fantasy. He became a legendary character on the streets during the past decade with theatrical flamboyancy, scabrous wit, and compelling charm. He was the grand master of push-and-pull, endearing one moment and scathingly critical the next.

When confined to his isolation room at Beth Israel Deaconess Medical Center last November after almost dying in the ICU, he dispatched me to the nearby Longwood Galleria with a detailed shopping list that included items from razors to pasta. When I returned an hour later and $30 poorer, he was so incensed by my choice of hair gels (CVS had only one kind!) that he was able to offer only the most begrudging thanks. Nonetheless, he dearly depended on our visits to him in the hospital, and each exasperated intern or resident would dutifully page (usually in the middle of the night) when he would refuse to consent to a needed test or emergency procedure until he had consulted "my private physician."

Many imponderables emerge from his story. For the last two years of his life, Brian had numerous prolonged stays at one or another of Boston's teaching hospitals—Boston Medical Center, Massachusetts General Hospital, Tufts Medical Center, Beth Israel Deaconess Medical Center, Lemuel Shattuck Hospital, or St. Elizabeth's Hospital. In between, he spent many months at McInnis House and four months in a nursing home. He routinely bounced back from death's doorstep, recovered much of his strength, and then returned to the streets—where he never lasted more than a week or so before the next hospital admission. On two occasions we arranged housing for him, once after several months at Barbara McInnis House and once after a prolonged admission to Shattuck Hospital, but he predictably fled to the streets at the eleventh hour. We puzzled over his fear of success, which always seemed to undermine his confidence and severely tested the mettle of his caregivers.

From February through July, following a harrowing admission to BMC, Brian was sent to a nursing home near Mattapan Square for hospice care. He rallied yet again—"I'm now on life #14"—and was granted an overnight pass in early August. He did not return and was found about a week later confused and very ill on the Esplanade along the Charles River at 4AM. He returned to the nursing home after a week at Massachusetts General Hospital, but the staff felt he was suicidal and too ill to manage and sent him to Boston Medical

Center. He was medically evaluated and sent back again to the nursing home. Within a day, the staff called 911 and had him sent to St. Elizabeth's Hospital for a "second opinion." After extensive medical and psychiatric testing, St. Elizabeth's attempted to have him return to the nursing home yet again. However, he was refused because he had become medically too complex for them to manage. We discussed the complicated situation with his doctors, who were clearly frustrated that the nursing home would not take him back. On Friday afternoon, we were nonplussed when Pine Street Inn called to let us know Brian was back at the shelter, having been discharged from the hospital without any scheduled medical follow-up despite his severe and advanced illness. I can only imagine the exasperation on all sides. Brian was too sick for a nursing home to handle but no longer required an expensive acute-care bed, but I could barely manage my anger with a system that would send this dying man to the streets on a weekend. I was also flabbergasted that, despite lengthy conversations with his doctors the previous day, no mention had been made of an impending discharge.

The van found him two nights later on the steps of St. Cecilia's Church near the corner of Massachusetts Avenue and Boylston Street. He was spitting angry with his disrupted care ("I'm sick of being a freakin' yo-yo!") and refused to consider either the hospital or Barbara McInnis House. He lasted a few more nights on the streets and finally called for help. The EMTs brought him to the emergency room at Boston Medical Center, where he showed us a deep leg wound that was infested with maggots. He seemed to improve over the following week or so, but when I stopped to see him the day I was leaving for vacation, pneumonia had swept through his lungs, and he was struggling for each breath. His last words to me: "Please don't leave." He died peacefully three days later. Our nurses Cheryl Kane and Sharon Morrison sat with him, placed lavender on his pillow, and took turns holding his hand. Toni Abraham, our new inpatient nurse practitioner, brought a tape of Brian's cherished ocean sounds to play in the background.

In sorting through some uncharacteristic anger toward a particular hospital, I realize that we all failed Brian, and I suspect we failed St. Elizabeth's Hospital rather than vice versa. Brian's journey over these past two years certainly chafes, and it underscores the importance of integrating homeless health care programs into the mainstream of the major teaching hospitals that provide much of the care to poor, vulnerable, and uninsured people in our cities. We are part of the system, and we need to own the dysfunction as well. The day I left for vacation, our street team had eighteen people inpatient at four different hospitals. This is the reality of the medical practice at BHCHP, and the quality and continuity of our care for individuals with so many acute and chronic medical and mental health illnesses are disproportionately dependent on hospital and specialty care.

The early vision remains vital and challenging: first, BHCHP as a "catalyst" within the mainstream health care system of Boston, a Trojan horse within each teaching hospital that releases a small cadre of clinicians into each institution's culture and practice, teaching each new generation of doctors and nurses to understand and address the special needs of those living without homes; second, BHCHP as a full participant in a city-wide service-delivery model that offers continuity of quality care and blurs the boundaries between shelters and hospitals, between medicine and public health, and between the medical, mental health, nursing, social work, and other clinical professions that are so used to working autonomously.

Lemuel Shattuck Hospital

DECEMBER 2001

A couple of weeks ago, I visited two stubborn rough sleepers who have been in the Lemuel Shattuck Hospital for the past few months. Charles Robinson, a 72-year-old man, had been sleeping in Boston Common directly down the hill from the State House last winter and spring. He literally tumbled out of his wheelchair onto the grass and collapsed each evening, sleeping through the extremes of weather and temperature until dawn.

His swollen legs festered, aggravated by urine draining down his tattered and way-too-short trousers, and precipitated multiple admissions to hospitals for cellulitis. Feisty and buoyed by a bevy of street friends living in Boston Common, he resisted all offers of assistance. He deteriorated rapidly over the summer, and his diabetes progressed untreated. We grew increasingly concerned about his health as well as his competence to care for himself. He was committed to the Neuro-Psychiatric Unit at the Shattuck Hospital in early July. During my visit I found a transformed character—ebullient, walking upright with a cane, absorbing the laughter and banter of a caring staff that teased and cajoled him. Happy and smiling, he told me he didn't miss Boston Common at all but wanted me to tell everyone there, "especially my girls," he was just dandy. His diabetes was under good control. However, the psychiatrist found him only moderately demented but capable of performing the basic activities of daily living. I shuddered. Interpretation: if he wanted to leave, no one would be able to hold him against his will. And then the cycle would begin all over again.

Edrick Carlyle, a Native American man legendary on Boston's streets and universally loved for his humor and gentle nature, had also been admitted to the same unit during the late summer after multiple admissions to New England Medical Center, which culminated in a life-threatening episode of "status epilepticus" (a prolonged and protracted seizure, threatening the oxygen supply to his brain). I found him childlike and bubbly as he recounted his daily routine of gym, cooking classes, and art therapy. In sixteen years I have never seen him radiate such joy. He was usually insensate and surrounded by vodka and Listerine bottles in his doorway on Arch Street.

His simplicity, due somewhat to an unrelenting sequence of seizures and head trauma over the years, was striking. He told me he had no interest in returning to the streets, and he had settled into the routine of the hospital and the company of friends and caring nurses and staff. The extraordinary care he has received is gratifying, and his response nothing short of miraculous. Yet, again, the psychiatrist explained that despite his limited mental capacity, he still was capa-

ble of the basic activities of daily living and could not be held against
his will any longer. He could feed himself, count his money, cross a
street. With the acute and sub-acute phase of his care completed, the
hospital was under considerable pressure to move him to a rest home
or nursing home for further care. However, he insists he will return
directly to the streets if he is not able to stay in the hospital. Change is
difficult and monumental for him, and he openly trembled when we
explored other possibilities. The contrast of his utter joy and comfort
within the rules and structure of the hospital against his somber and
withdrawn life drinking and sleeping on the sidewalks for two decades
is hard to fathom while chatting with him in the hospital cafeteria.
Yet now the hospital is faced with an impossible but all-too-familiar
dilemma. He is well enough to no longer need costly acute and sub-
acute care, and a safe discharge to a nursing home is now imminent.
Yet if he refuses (or cannot tolerate) a transfer or if no nursing homes
with available beds will accept him, he will be discharged to the streets
and will be back on the sidewalk in front of St. Anthony's Shrine on
Arch Street near Downtown Crossing. During the past years, he has
logged countless emergency room visits and hospitalizations with
many prolonged ICU stays. If he is discharged to the streets, the pat-
tern of costly utilizations of health care and other services will recur,
jeopardizing these four months of intense intervention.

He had spent over five years in the Vermont Youth Center as a
juvenile, but he had been on Boston's streets for almost two decades.
His mother, a wonderful woman whom we cared for many years ago,
died on the streets at the age of 42.

Visiting these two men who are now thriving after many years of
unwavering efforts by so many was a lesson in patience and resilience.
Such transformations remind us to never give up the hope that the
seemingly impossible can be achieved. In the routine of our daily
lives caring for people who have endured such trauma and poverty,
success is often incremental and infinitesimal. The limits of the ability of these two men to choose good options and to care adequately for themselves casts the issue of civil liberties into stark relief. I

must confess that I would have been jubilant if the psychiatrist had declared both incompetent and unable to return to the streets, but I reluctantly accept that the law errs deliberately on the side of protecting civil liberties.

Listening
MARCH 2002

During intense discussions about vision
and organization this past week, the
nagging but critical issue of "quality"
emerged as pivotal in parsing BHCHP's
simple but deceptively difficult mission
statement: to provide or assure the
highest quality health care for homeless
men, women, and children in Boston.
The benchmarks, milestones, outcome
measures, critical pathways, and
the host of other mandates of plans
and insurers are clearly necessary,
and we will continue to work feverishly
to provide the best in health care
for our patients.

But these do not inspire us as clinicians, and they fail to capture the core of BHCHP or the essence of the doctor- (read: nurse practitioner-, physician assistant-, or nurse-) patient relationship. Reflections on that relationship, an ancient covenant, render such descriptions as clients, consumers, customers, service utilizers, and "covered lives" anathema.

Roger Ramsey, despite his youthful 43 years, ranks among the most difficult, contrary, cantankerous, and outrageous individuals I have encountered in these seventeen years of caring for homeless persons. A proud denizen of the streets, he is curt, combative, and vituperative. His nightly badgering of the van staff includes an expletive-laden recitation of the litany of shelters and soup kitchens from which he has been banned. The stories behind each ban would make your hair stand on end. His approach to the world is explosive and confrontational, and he rages loudly about the "lousy hand" he has been dealt in life. He belittles health care workers for "never listening," even though he frequently presents with a plethora of somatic complaints which result in exhaustive and futile evaluations.

A loner from New Bedford, he couldn't sit still in school and couldn't calm an inner rage. He fought constantly and stood up to everyone, but he was more often pummeled than victorious. He was on the streets by age seventeen, quelling his inner storm with a host of substances, finding trouble brewing in most alleys and doorways, and beginning a longstanding joust with the courts and prisons. When I first met him in 1986, he mentioned that the only time he felt in control was in a prison cell—usually solitary confinement given his issues with authority.

In the early 1990s, he bought a bus ticket to the West Coast but bailed out in Las Vegas. Gambling, the desert, and a city that never sleeps captivated him. He suffered a devastating leg injury while hitchhiking, with multiple fractures necessitating several surgical procedures and much hardware in the ensuing years. He scrambled back to Boston and arrived with an infection deep in the bones of the shattered leg. Despite exhaustive efforts, this osteomyelitis never truly healed. Two years ago we faced a difficult decision together: either amputate the leg above the knee or place a rod that would fuse the leg and prevent Roger from ever bending his knee again. He chose the latter and came to McInnis House for post-operative care.

"Go ahead, laugh. I know I'm a useless peg leg now!"

He lasted a few weeks, until he smashed the pay phone and threatened the staff. I had never known him to leave any place voluntarily; he somehow needed to be barred or expelled as a way of deflecting any responsibility.

Whenever Roger came to the clinic, he would storm in with a list of immediate demands. He constantly badgered us for more pain medication, which was difficult to manage given his alcohol and drug use. He was convinced we were not hearing his complaints, and he protested boisterously.

"No one ever listens to me! Give me the damn pills and I won't have to drink or score drugs."

We negotiated through several broken medication contracts, arranged innumerable detoxification beds, and generally felt as if we were treading water with this complicated man. As we got to know him better, we saw a gentle and wounded soul come through the angry and threatening veneer. He would laugh with us, joke about current events, compliment, and even offer muffled thanks to the nurses.

On the streets, his leg never healed and the infection persisted, giving him intense pain that he treated with a smorgasbord of substances. During one of his famed and self-named "hissy fits" in Downtown Crossing about a year ago, the police apprehended him and held him in protective custody. He had some outstanding warrants and ended up with two years to serve in South Bay House of Corrections. Several of the warrants were for urinating in public. Roger grumbled that the charges for public urination were now called "exposure." With three such charges, he was considered a low-level sex offender.

Once incarcerated, prisoners' health care is assumed by the corrections health system. I felt sheepishly guilty but frankly relieved that someone else would have to deal with Roger's outbursts and demands for a while. Constant and bitter complaints of intense back pain, by a man who had cried wolf too much, fell on skeptical and deaf ears. He began to write long letters from his isolation cell, and while I enjoyed them immensely, I trusted the system and fully understood this classic "difficult patient." The letters kept coming, asking for John Grisham books, a subscription to the Boston Herald, and, ever more urgently, help with his pain. He couldn't sleep, and prolonged sitting or standing caused severe pain in his lower back that radiated down the length of his right leg. This was new and very worrisome to me, as his innumerable surgeries and chronic pain had been in the left leg, never the right.

After cutting through the usual red tape, we visited him on Halloween. He had been incarcerated six months and was a gaunt shadow of his former blustery and cocky self. His skin was blanched and diaphoretic, his loss of weight dramatic, and his months of agony became horrifyingly apparent. The lung cancer, present but not noticed on his admission chest x-ray to jail, had metastasized and crushed six of the bones in his spine. An MRI done a few months earlier had revealed compression fractures in his vertebrae, but the results had not been communicated to the prison medical staff. Our pleas were as hollow as the echoes of the cell doors closing, and the ways of the prison system as arcane as you have seen in many Hollywood films. Roger did receive palliative radiation therapy at BMC for the compression fractures of his spine over the ensuing six weeks, but his abhorrence of the corrections system spewed forth in his animated refusal to consider admission to the Shattuck Hospital for chemotherapy.

Roger's prognosis was grave, maybe a few months at best. We pushed hard for parole, which he was granted in early January. But the bureaucracy stalled; parole requires both internal and external review. The volume of letters escalated as his health deteriorated. He was admitted to Boston Medical Center with shortness of breath caused by an aspiration pneumonia. The cancer in his lung had grown large enough to block his esophagus, and he had difficulty swallowing food. Stubborn, angry, and resilient, he kept eating whatever he wanted when he returned to prison.

I was on the van around midnight when the ICU physician called me on February 6. Roger, still chained to his bed and accompanied by two prison guards, was struggling for air. He refused a breathing machine when we couldn't guarantee that he would get better. We called his brother in New Bedford. He was instructed to go to South Bay for "clearance" before he could enter the hospital room of his shackled and dying brother. As his doctor, I could freely see him, so I never thought to tell his brother to go first to the prison at 2AM!

Roger defied the odds and lived from Wednesday until early Sunday morning. Besides our staff, only his beloved brother came to see him. As always, Sharon Morrison, our nurse, was remarkable, massaging his feet, bathing and turning his emaciated body, and keeping lavender on his pillow. I spent many late hours in his room, relieving his exhausted brother while cherishing these last conversations with a man who so fascinated and confused me.

His single request of me was to not let him die in chains. Heroic efforts by Sarah Ciambrone and Barry Bock convinced the external parole board to free him on Friday evening, as long as we promised that McInnis House would be his post-release address, a requirement for parole. (Interestingly, those who complete or wrap their sentences and have no parole are allowed to go directly to the streets and shelters.) The chains were removed, the uniformed guards departed, and Roger finally gave up his struggle and found some peace. I was with him when he died early Sunday morning. His last words to me:

"I told you no one ever listens. But thanks."

With some unease, I found myself sharing in his rage—indignant at a system that ignored his pain, made him a number, chained him to his deathbed, and frankly missed a crucial diagnosis. Death tendered a fleeting glimpse into the lifelong fury of a man dealt an unplayable hand, born with dreams dashed and opportunities limited by a chemistry that bathed him in pain and anger. But his stunning courage and rare honesty emerged unscathed. To the end he remained his own person.

Lost Treasure

AUGUST 2003

I was in Rhode Island when the page from Barbara McInnis came just after 1AM last Friday morning, a few hours before she died and left us devastated. I have been hardwired to respond posthaste to pages from Barbara ever since she first introduced me to the Pine Street Nurses' Clinic eighteen years ago and tutored me in the health care of homeless people.

Barbara usually calls to seek help for others—homeless persons, friends in need of hospital care, or urgent medical consultations—or to urge me to advocate on behalf of persons who have been treated poorly in our city's health care system. I am among the legion constitutionally unable to say no to Barbara. I remember a Friday night call many years ago when a man from Africa had arrived at Pine Street Inn and was in severe heart failure from a faulty aortic valve:

"Jim, he needs to get to Brigham and Women's Hospital right away for surgery. He has no money, no insurance, and no USA citizenship, but he needs our help. Please try your best to arrange this."

The task took days, but the hospital and the cardiac surgery team were extraordinary. He had successful open-heart surgery a week later.

The call from her hospital bed in Maine was different. She had been a passenger in her partner Kathy's car several days ago in Portland when they were blindsided by a drunk driver. She underwent successful surgery to repair the compound fracture of the femur in her right leg. But tonight she had awakened in her hospital bed markedly short of breath, and she could barely finish a sentence during our conversation. She wanted to know why, and we talked about some possibilities, all of which were worrisome to me: pneumonia, sepsis, pulmonary embolus, fat embolus, heart failure. She asked if I would call her doctors and talk with them. I promised but urged her to alert the nurses of her symptoms immediately, even though I knew she did not want to bother them at this early hour. I called the nurses' station on her floor and spoke with the charge nurse, who told me that the covering physician had already been notified and was on her way to evaluate Barbara. She was reluctant to give me any more information without Barbara's written permission. I pointed out that Barbara never complained and that I was sure something very, very serious had happened for which urgent help was needed. I received a perfunctory thank you and assurance that everything would be fine.

Several years ago while visiting friends in England, I stumbled upon Theodore Zeldin's book, *An Intimate History of Humanity*. Unbeknownst to me, the author had made a journey to America to gather information, had interviewed Barbara, and had captured her magic and essence in a few brief sentences:

"I make no plans. I have no dream of a different society. I never think about that. I'm busy surviving, like the guests. I am intuitive... we are overwhelmed."

She worked quietly and exhaustively, helping those most in need, never seeking office or honor or position. While she may not have dreamed of a different society, the lives of myself and countless others have been forever changed by her generosity and tender mercy.

Barbara is the only true saint I've ever known: funny, loving, brilliant, frumpy, gentle, irascible, wise, humble, stubborn, and unpredictable. As we used to marvel while watching *Miami Vice* every Friday night after clinic, Barbara was dynamically present to the Cosmic Unfolding. She was always herself, whether talking with dignitaries such as Mother Teresa, comforting those suffering under a bridge or down a dark alley, or regaling us with stories at Doyle's Pub. The soul of Boston's inner city, Barbara was trusted by homeless people and revered throughout the local and national health care for the homeless community.

Barbara has been my mentor, muse, friend, and conscience since the day our program began in 1985. Barbara deftly deflected all praise and every honor, and I was never as proud as the day McInnis House opened in 1993 when Barbara too beamed with pride alongside her mother and family.

Barbara drilled us on the basics incessantly and relentlessly. The core of the healing art is the personal relationship. Doctors and nurse practitioners and physician assistants need to leave the traditional clinics and venture out to join the nurses in places familiar to persons living in shelters and on the streets. Seek every opportunity to share food or coffee, be present in the lives of others, and listen to their stories. Offer care and relieve suffering, never judge. We are not in the business of changing people; our purpose is to gently offer hope and options. Barbara's wisdom and compassion have always been the heart and soul of our program.

The death of Barbara McInnis is still too fresh to comprehend. She lived life in abundance and called out the very best in each of us. We have been blessed by her presence and enjoined to embrace the care of those forgotten or ignored by society and by our health care institutions.

Barbara sought justice and eschewed charity. When she first went to Pine Street Inn in the early 1970s, she insisted on getting paid. She gave money to homeless folks only on Sundays. When BHCHP began, she insisted that we employ doctors and that we not use volunteers. She told me that first night that I needed to stick with this job, that consistency and continuity were as important as my medical skills. I would have to carry my beeper so that homeless persons could call me whenever I was needed, whatever the hour. I cherish the memory of that 1AM call when she needed me during those last hours of her truly magnificent life.

Homeless Haunts

MARCH 2005

After receiving my fifteenth letter from prison from one of our more animated and engaging street persons, I journeyed to Norfolk State Prison last night and found that I had to complete a lengthy form and wait for five business days before I could be "cleared" to visit him. I last visited George Garrison in early January when he was still being held at the Nashua Street Jail. He angrily lamented on the telephone across some very thick glass that he had been arrested as a suspect in what later proved to be a case of mistaken identity.

I am embarrassed to admit that I actually understood the detectives'
conundrum when they arrested him, as I know the real murder suspect well, and George looks eerily similar. Unfortunately, and in a
quite common scenario, the arrest triggered a search for outstanding
warrants, and George is now incarcerated for several minor offenses
that occurred about five years ago in Quincy.

I have received many letters from prison over the years. Raw and
bare-bones, void of ego and self-pity, these letters emerge from the
depths and offer a compelling glimpse into the struggle to find hope
amidst failure, confinement, and isolation. I remember my capti-
vation during the late 1960s with the startling prison reflections of
Dietrich Bonhoeffer just before his execution for complicity in the
failed Munich plot to assassinate Hitler. While not literary in the
classical sense, George's letters are no less a *cri de coeur* and depict a
journey into chaos and desperation. He vacillates from born again
to bitter social critic, meanders from childish longings to profound
insight, and reflects on a life of poverty and deprivation punctuated
by all-too-brief moments of passion and joy. He seeks some shred of
meaning and purpose, some hope that he can make a difference to
someone, somewhere, sometime.

George Garrison is a proud former Marine who never saw action
in a war. Born in Boston City Hospital, the fourteenth of fifteen children, he grew up in the restive Charlestown projects at the foot of
Bunker Hill. He has a vivid memory from age five of seeing his father
die of a brain hemorrhage at home on the same day that President
Kennedy was assassinated. His mother died six years later of meta-
static cancer after a long illness, during which he and two brothers
were placed in foster care. He recalls how his foster parents called the
brothers into the living room and told them their mother had died.

"That was the turning point. Everything went downhill from
there."

The foster home was strict and often violent, and George frequently ran away, regularly hiding in the basement of a friend for weeks. He
was taken in by an alcoholic sister who lived above a bar until an older

brother brought fifteen-year-old George to live with him and work on a farm in Idaho. He did well in school but began drinking and experimenting with marijuana and LSD. He left high school when he turned eighteen to join the Marines. After Camp Pendleton, he was stationed near San Diego, CA. He was stateside his entire two years.

"I was a grunt and proud as hell. Our platoon was always first in the marching drills. But I never saw any action, and I kept drinking. I loved going to Tijuana and Los Angeles on the weekends. I never got in any trouble, and I have an honorable discharge."

He headed to Portland and tried to stay sober, but he alternated between the streets and incarcerations for forgery, assault and battery, and drunk and disorderly conduct. He met his future wife in 1980, worked in telemarketing and fund-raising, and managed to stay clean and sober for over a decade. He relapsed, began selling cocaine to support his habit, and sustained serious head trauma when he was assaulted with a baseball bat in 1993. Two months later he began having seizures, and his behavior became erratic with wide mood swings and explosive outbursts. He managed to keep working, but he recounts coming home one evening in 1994 to find his wife in bed with his best friend.

"I walked out the door, got on a Greyhound bus, drank a bottle of whiskey, and came directly back to Boston. I was devastated, and the pain has never gone away."

Except for a brief two-week job in Framingham, George has been on the streets of Boston for this past decade. He often spends time in the South Bay or Dedham jails for non-violent crimes, usually check forgery, his "specialty" on the streets. His longest period of incarceration has been six months, and he spends his prison days in the library, reading and writing letters.

"I'm usually the only one in the library. I was there when bin Laden leveled the World Trade Centers and wanted to bust out and go find the creep. I was there when the Democratic National Convention came to Boston and regretted that I couldn't be out there to help protect folks."

George cannot sleep at night because of nightmares and "crazy" fears. He has flashbacks of the deaths of his parents, of incessant whippings with a leather belt, of jailhouse fights when he couldn't back down and ended up with broken noses and facial bones. He has fears that someone is behind him and about to attack him. He panhandles on Lansdowne Street outside Fenway Park during the baseball season and on Causeway Street near Boston Garden when the Bruins or Celtics are playing. He always holds up the same cardboard sign: "Hit me in the stomach as hard as you can for $1 or in the face for $5."

I saw him several times in Nashua Street, and I later journeyed four times to the prison in Dedham in the median of Route 128 but was always thwarted by red tape and never managed to visit with him. On my last attempt to visit, I arrived at 6PM to be processed as instructed. The visiting times for George were limited to Tuesdays and Saturdays from 6:15PM to 7PM. I waited dutifully until 7PM, when the guard informed me that George had been sent to Quincy Court earlier in the day, and the van had not yet returned. I was summarily dismissed. The next night on the van we found George sober and somber on the streets. He was thrilled that the judge had been impressed with his good behavior but then dismayed to be released directly to the streets. George cherished the structure of life in jail ("23 hours a day in my cell, three meals, no cigarettes") and was genuinely upset to be back on the streets with no money and five months of fragile sobriety. He had been working with the Salvation Army in Saugus to enter a long-term recovery program, and he had thoroughly expected to be sent there directly from prison. This interlude on the street was not planned. Since the temperature was fifteen degrees, we brought him to Barbara McInnis House to try and connect him to a program.

George is a staunch defender of civil rights and of his comrades on the streets. His letters almost always advocate passionately for equality and justice. While at McInnis House, he wrote a letter to his fellow patients who were disgruntled over a new rule.

A Note I Wrote

We here at the McInnis House are Homeless for a reason whether it be because of Personal Losses, Unemployment, Divorce, Drug and Alcohol Addiction, lack of Job Skills, Head Trauma. Whatever it may be, there is a reason.

We are here to take care of our Medical Issues, to get well and start thinking with a clear head, which in some of us is a very hard thing to do, but we are faced now with a 50-50, meaning to go back to the streets where people are getting robbed, beat up, or murdered more than ever. We are all vulnerable targets on the streets, and we mind this opportunity to avoid this unnecessary life on the streets. This is the decision we are offered here at McInnis House. Most of the staff here are beautiful in heart. They can and do put themselves in our shoes and most don't care about their paychecks. The most important thing to them is us as individuals. The staff cares for us so much that they take time to talk with us individually to get to know us better, our needs, and plans. From my experience this is the only place of its kind in the United States. They don't look at us as Homeless Haunts, but as real individuals with needs. They put us in programs if that's what we need or want. They help us with personal needs, Housing, SSDI, SSI, Food Stamps. Whatever our individual needs are they put 150% in to help us accomplish our endeavors in a positive fashion.

So let's all of us be very thankful and more respectful to these most caring and unbelievable staff members who are here to help us. So please let's be more honest and open and respectful to these people. They are one of a kind. Some homeless people will never get this opportunity. So please let's all take advantage of this blessing and realize what is best for us. Thank you for listening and GOD BLESS all of you.

George Garrison

P.S. Please remember that in this life no one is better than anyone else. We are all related and created of equalness, no matter what race, creed, or color, in one way or the other. Thank you.

George is unsettled, no longer willing to look for a recovery program, and desperate for housing. The weather has been improving, and he has been ornery, persnickety, and bitter. I recognize this behavior as a sign that he feels the call of the streets. I have no doubt he will soon abscond, and we all try to keep him from feeling ashamed or guilty.

Springtime Hopes

MAY 2005

The renovation of the Mallory Institute
of Pathology and the emerging
capital campaign have proven stern
taskmasters, caulking just about every
fault and crack in our calendars.
Cheryl Kane, our street-team nurse
for years, has taken on the challenge
of raising the millions of needed
dollars; she is assisted by Linda
Wood-O'Connor, whom we shamelessly
stole from Pine Street Inn and the
Jesuits. Our board refers to them
as the "hold-up twins" because they
are so genuine and gentle that
saying no is impossible.

Meetings this week with our senior management and with the architects have focused us on the interesting challenges and unique opportunities that loom on the rapidly approaching horizon. Form and function are subtly merging as we confront the dynamic and inescapable interplay between mission/vision and the design of this new space. For example, the exciting new clinic offers sufficient exam and clinic rooms to integrate, within several "pods," medicine and mental health with nursing and case management, and it also creates new possibilities for the teaching and education of students and residents. The design of clinical "pods" assumes a shared vision of our practice model; a multitude of similar design issues for respite, office, and other space has been the genesis of much excitement within our program. As the Chinese proverb says, may you live in interesting times.

In the early nineteenth century, the famed physician and pathologist Virchow noted "doctors are often called to be the lawyers for the poor." While this is no longer true, thanks to Sarah Anderson and the many lawyers willing to work for legal services or devote *pro bono* time to those in need, disability entitlements remain an intriguing holdover. Despite my pride in the excellent care we offer our patients, I have come to acknowledge that assisting homeless persons through the disability process is often the most effective health care intervention we can offer. For those who meet the criteria for this entitlement, an income and health insurance are forthcoming, frequently paving the sole avenue to escape homelessness. We have worked closely with the National Health Care for the Homeless Council and the Social Security Administration (SSA) to train physicians and other clinicians in the navigation of the murky disability documentation process.

Doctors have been the major problem, from my perspective. There is at most a paltry payment of $25 for the hours of work involved, which is deplorable. But more importantly, we do not understand the process, speak and write in a whole different language, and frankly have neither the training nor the time to efficiently complete the letters requested by our patients. Salvation can sometimes be found in a tome called the *Listing of Impairments*, which translates federal hieroglyphics into barely recognizable medical *patois*, at least enough to make the process less arcane. David Buchanan, a remarkable colleague of ours at Cook County Hospital in Chicago, where doctors are barraged with requests for these letters, found that over 80% of the physicians there had never heard of the *Listing of Impairments*. Since the requirements for disability are carefully delineated under each medical or mental health problem in this book, these doctors are undoubtedly frustrated by the futility of completing complex forms and submitting the necessary letters. I could go on, but suffice it to say I was surprised by the turnout at our training sessions in several cities across the country. While the topic remains a decided soporific, the growing interest among doctors in helping the poor in their clinics has been startling and gratifying.

Despite the grandiosity of the above paragraphs, I remain humbly aware that the ridiculous trumps the sublime most of the time. Life on the streets, on the van, and at McInnis House keeps us humble and grounded in stark realities. Poverty is still the most overwhelming social determinant of health, a fact which dwarfs our effectiveness as doctors and healers. My visits to McInnis House are bedrock. The cinderblocks on a granite slab notwithstanding, the place has a unique warmth and vitality that contrast sharply with the raw edges of life on the streets. The realization usually catches us by surprise: walking into the lobby at 9PM to hear the explosion of cheers as David Ortiz hits a grand slam; listening to conversations in the back patio on topics ranging from the new Pope to leaks in the Big Dig to sincere concerns for friends still outside; or seizing a few moments to share a cup of coffee and just catch up. Some of my fondest memories come from weekend and evening conversations sitting with our patients on the benches in the back patio.

Last night the nurses had asked me to stop by and help allay the escalating anxiety of Ralph Emilio, who has end-stage liver failure from hepatitis C and alcohol, and who is desperately hoping to qualify for a liver transplant. The waiting list is long, the evaluation arduous, and his chaotic life over the past twenty years renders him a very poor candidate. Candidly cognizant of the consequences of his own behavior, he also understands that he is facing death without the transplant. In the best of times, this man is frenetic. He is perhaps the most anxious and restless person I've ever known, but the stress of his illness has catapulted his anxiety into the stratosphere. The nurses are remarkably tolerant of his behavior, and surprisingly the other patients sense his desperation and are also very kind and tolerant. Ralph finds some consolation after we call his twin brother, who had a liver and kidney transplant five years ago, and who is now thriving in their hometown of Hartford, Connecticut. But as with so many who have lived on the streets for decades, Ralph's seven siblings remain supportive but too scarred by past failures to get involved at this time.

Our favorite Red Sox fan and long-term McInnis House patient Joe Firestone moved into a wonderful apartment in Maverick Square last Friday. Joe's claim to the Barbara McInnis House "Hall of Fame" is that he spent six of his last seven birthdays there; most recently he had been there for almost two years as we abandoned hope of discharging him without a safe place to go. Upon every previous discharge to the shelter or streets, he was in the ICU within days because of his very severe and advanced lung disease and his inability to stay sober in those environments. Sarah Ciambrone and the McInnis House staff have been stellar in their creative care for this very special man, who first hit the streets when he ran away from home at age thirteen and hitchhiked from Worcester to Phoenix. Our team has been visiting him twice a week in his new home on the East Boston waterfront in an effort to keep him safe and out of the emergency room. Sarah has arranged for him to come to Barbara McInnis House twice a week to work in the clothing room, and he now spends two days a week working on his GED. While it's too early to tell, we are hoping that he will defy all the odds and finally end his 30 years of living on the streets.

The Bigelow

JULY 2005

I spent June as the visiting physician on the Bigelow Medical Service at Massachusetts General Hospital. The month was demanding, exhilarating, and exhausting. Combing through the remnants of neglected stuff on my desk and computer screen, I am once again paralyzed by the relentless tyranny of e-mail, wading through way too many unopened and unanswered missives. But I'm honestly grateful for a wondrous month immersed in medicine, teaching and learning with the interns and residents, sharing thoughts with specialists, and caring for inpatients. The pace of change in medicine has accelerated dramatically, and the need to stay abreast is ever more urgent.

Homelessness is woven into the fabric of daily life on the Massachusetts General Hospital wards. McInnis House, rarely spelled correctly and often confused with the Irish stout, has crept into the vernacular on daily rounds. The obstacles to care presented by homelessness are magnified on the inpatient wards, where information is instantly available, tests and procedures performed posthaste, and home services efficiently arranged at discharge. Homelessness grinds the wheels to a halt, with histories tough to piece together, information scattered across the city and state, and safe discharge planning options limited.

About 20% of the individuals admitted to our service came directly from the shelters or the streets—not appreciably different from years past. The acuity, severity, and complexity of the illnesses can be dramatic. Michael Crichton, while a third-year student at Harvard Medical School, wrote a short book called *Five Patients* about his experience on the medical wards at MGH; the long shadow cast by his 6'8" frame notwithstanding, let me share the brief stories of five homeless persons admitted to our service during June.

A 35-year-old man seen frequently by BHCHP's HIV and Street Teams was sent directly from Nashua Street Jail with an alteration in mental status, bizarre behavior that in retrospect had led to his arrest a few days earlier. We struggled to find a cause for his confusion and delirium. He was immune-compromised with advanced AIDS and a very low CD4 cell count, making him vulnerable to opportunistic infections of the brain and nervous system. Lethargic and minimally responsive, he looked gravely ill. An electroencephalogram (EEG) showed that he was seizing continuously, a condition called status epilepticus. A diagnostic MRI could not be done because he has bullet fragments in his neck and spine from an old gunshot wound. We sent him to the ICU for intubation and induction of a phenobarbital coma to control the seizures and minimize the damage to his brain cells. Anti-retroviral treatment for his AIDS was rapidly initiated, but his kidneys collapsed as a side effect of one of the medications, and he required emergent hemodialysis. After two weeks in this induced coma, his kidneys began to open up, and his seizures became quiescent. Subsequent studies showed marked abnormalities in his brain that were the likely foci of his seizures. These abnormalities could be due to an infection (toxoplasmosis is the most likely) or to lymphoma. The treatment for each of these is markedly different, and a biopsy of this area of the brain is usually necessary to distinguish between the two. Such an invasive procedure was deemed too risky, and by the end of the month we still had no clear answers.

I had met this man many times in the past on our street and van rounds. He was aloof, elusive, and proud. On the streets we had no luck in engaging him in care. I was surprised when his family came to visit him from New York City, and his sister exulted that he had graduated from college with a degree in chemistry. Her husband is a very prominent doctor in the South Bronx who specializes in HIV.

This man's roommate was a 43-year-old individual whom we have known for years on the streets. He sleeps in an ATM on Tremont Street, and he never seeks care or asks us for help. He occasionally accepts food and blankets from the van, but he proudly refuses any further assistance. His neck and back grew intensely painful during the last weeks of May, and he finally sought help in the MGH emergency room in early June. He exchanged some regrettable words with a nurse, and the security guards escorted him out of the hospital and back to Cambridge Street. The pain worsened, and, remorseful and barely able to walk, he returned a day later. He had a high fever, and a CT scan showed abscesses in both lungs, in the lining of his lungs and heart, and in the epidural space around his spinal cord. His body was riddled with methicillin-resistant *Staphylococcus aureus* (the notorious MRSA that made the cover of *Time* not long ago), and he was rushed to the ICU for intubation and the placement of two chest tubes to drain the fluid around his lungs. Two days later he underwent neurosurgery to stabilize his spine from the neck to the mid-back. A few days later he came to our floor with tubes in both lungs and drains from his neck, bladder, and the left paraspinous muscle where more pus had been found. His spirit was indomitable, and he improved slowly on a cocktail of strong antibiotics and surprisingly little pain medication. His mother came from New Bedford to visit, and she cried as she told us about the travails he suffered as a slow learner who was mercilessly taunted by schoolmates. Cocaine calmed him down, alcohol boosted his self-esteem, and he began a three-decade sojourn on the streets of Providence and Boston. He confessed to me one morning that his fall from a twenty-foot overpass last September was really "a deliberate swan dive." He spent months at Rhode Island Hospital recovering from shattered bones and a lacerated liver and spleen.

Across the hall, entrenched for the entire month with no options for a safe discharge, was another long-time patient of ours. Years of seething anger had erupted from this 45-year-old man as he struggled with cirrhosis and end-stage liver disease. Barred from every shelter in town as well as the Boston Night Center and Barbara McInnis House (a rare trifecta in our world), he had been jettisoned from two nursing homes for insolence, drug use, and threatening behavior. Docile and contrite with us, he was grateful to be inside and safe. He became more yellow and jaundiced with each passing day, and a liver biopsy finally established that cancer was destroying what was left of his severely damaged liver. No family or visitors ever came to see him during the month of June. On the window near his bed were pictures of a woman with two beautiful daughters. I would catch him staring longingly, but he turned gruff when I asked him questions and simply said they didn't exist for him anymore.

A 55-year-old man with severe diabetes and infections in several toes was sent to MGH from McInnis House with a high fever. He was a patient whom our team had been seeing for over a decade on the streets, usually near Carson Beach in South Boston. He rarely went in to the shelters and proudly boasted about surviving every snowstorm this past harsh winter. His nasty disposition served as a weapon to keep people at bay. His relationships with women on the streets were passionate and often violent. His partner of many years, a delightful young woman from Duxbury on the South Shore, froze to death in January of 2004 in a field near Andrew Station. Although he was not with her at the time of her tragic death (the day before, she had left the ICU at Boston Medical Center against medical advice (AMA) during an admission for profound hypothermia), he has been wracked with guilt ever since. His diabetes was complicated by a dense peripheral neuropathy, leaving him without feeling in either foot. As a consequence he had already lost a toe to frostbite, and he had neglected enlarging ulcers on the soles of both feet. Upon admission to our floor, the infection had spread into the bones and now required six weeks of antibiotics. Because of a complication in the treatment, he needed to be off all antibiotics for two weeks prior to a critical bone biopsy, which would help establish the offending organism and guide our choice of antibiotic. We sent him back to Barbara McInnis House for this two-week period, avoiding a prolonged and costly stay in the hospital, since he was not eligible for nursing home or skilled nursing care during that period. He has done very well there, and he will have his bone biopsy in the next ten days.

Finally, an 80-year-old man who has been on the streets of various cities in America for the past four decades was admitted with heart failure. I met him ten years ago when I was on street rounds at South Station, where he spent most of his days reading books. He declined my offer of a cup of coffee and insisted on Earl Grey tea. We sat and chatted for a while, and he was excited to learn that I was a philosophy major in college. That began a weekly tradition of meeting for tea, reviewing the *New York Times* headlines, and discussing world events. All inquiries about his own life were deflected. He began to spend most nights at the Night Center, where I would look forward to seeing him on Wednesdays. He kept to himself, was suspicious of the other guests, and was fiercely territorial about the corner of the room where he would sit and occasionally sleep. One night he proudly announced that he had been the youngest person ever to teach at Columbia University, his *alma mater*. He graduated at the age of 16, and he was classmates and friends with a slew of American icons, including Allan Ginsberg, Jack Kerouac, and Lucien Carr. Two of his devoted mentors, Mark Van Doren and Lionel Trilling, were giants in the world of literature and philosophy whom I had read and admired while in college. My skepticism led me to ask questions about the latter, and he gave colorful details of their style in the classroom and their penchant for cigars and port.

"Certain things happened and I was persecuted by those who were jealous of my success."

He would not discuss this further other than to say that his parents gave him a trust fund and sent him to wander through Europe for five years during the dark days of the McCarthy era. He came back to New York disgruntled, and after President Kennedy's assassination he grew convinced of a plot to kill or imprison him. He fled New York City and began a 40-year pilgrimage through paranoia and through innumerable towns and shelters across America.

He finally agreed to come to see me at our MGH Street Clinic, only two blocks from the Night Center. Despite Herculean efforts to win his trust and confidence, he refused to accept any "doctoring." He would come into the examination room to discuss philosophy and literature—and to garner a meal ticket for our cafeteria. He resolutely refused even to have his blood pressure checked. I learned to schedule my visits with him over the lunch break so that I could enjoy the unencumbered time with him. He was a voracious reader with a steel-trap memory, and he never failed to fascinate. I have always been interested in Jack Kerouac, who was a native of Lowell and a star high-school football player there. When I asked about Jack, he frowned and dashed my excitement.

"I met him several times with Allan Ginsberg. A dashing young man for sure, but a terribly shallow thinker."

His impeccable manners and eloquent speech contrasted with his disheveled and noisome appearance. With much cajoling, he had once come to McInnis House for a shower and a few days of "rest," and he treated us all with magnificent piano recitals. Two episodes of life-threatening arrhythmias left him short of breath and caused damage to his fragile heart. On each occasion he had come to the emergency room but had refused to be admitted to the hospital and would not accept any medication. Near the end of May he came to our Thursday Street Clinic breathless and ashen with massively swollen feet. His spirit had been broken when he realized he could neither walk up the flight of stairs to the Night Center nor negotiate the several steps to his occasional room in a Brookline inn. Exhausted and very ill, he agreed to come into the hospital from the clinic that day so we could treat his severe heart failure. He remains in the hospital, too weak and too depressed to flee. I visited him most evenings during the month to absorb my daily infusion of philosophy. In his private room are three flowers brought to him by Jeanne Marie, one of our Street Clinic volunteers. He cherishes these flowers and has refused to let the staff throw the now wilting and blackened roses away.

The images on the following pages were taken by John Baynard. John has worked as a documentary filmmaker for 30 years. He has been cameraman on a wide range of documentaries, including *Murder on the Rio San Juan* (Frontline), *Don King Unauthorized* (Frontline), *My Mother's Murder* (HBO), and *Sister Aimee* (American Experience). www.johnbaynard.com ▶

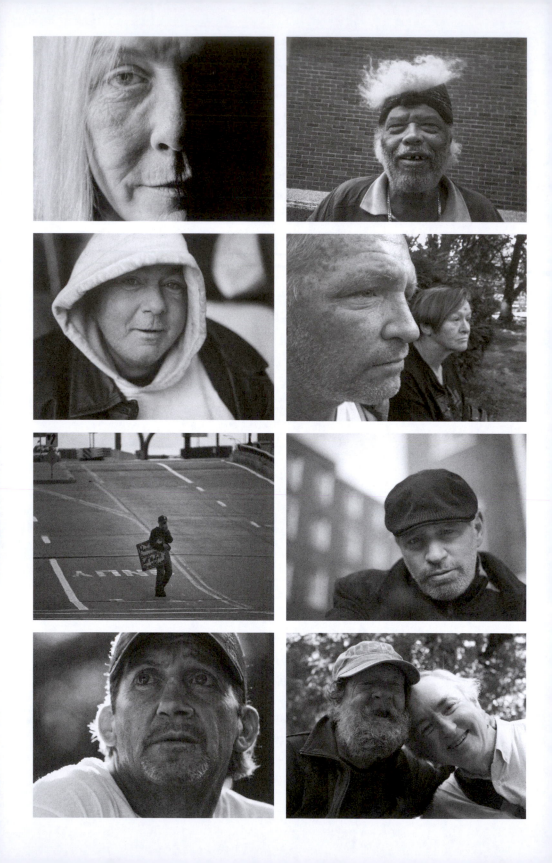

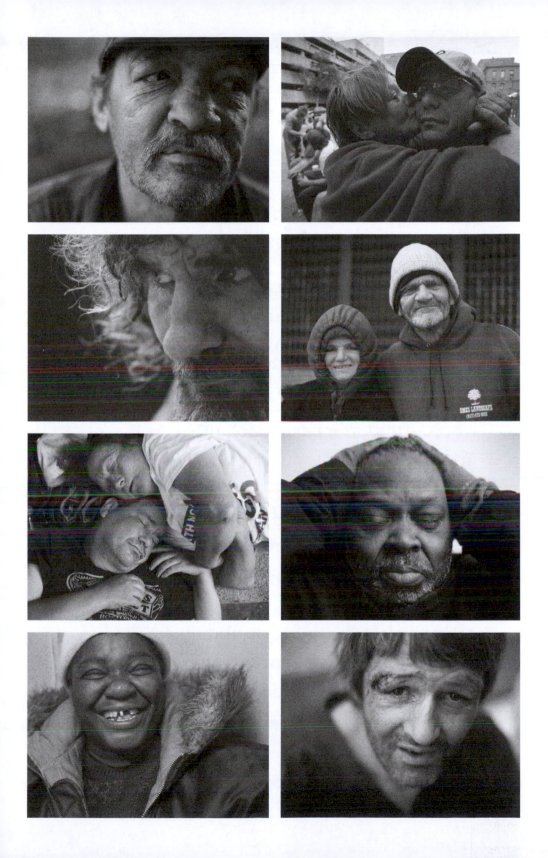

Urban Prophets

MARCH 2006

On a cold January evening last winter
we gathered in the basement of St.
Anthony's Shrine on Arch Street
in the heart of downtown Boston
to remember Malcolm Norbert, a
49-year-old Air Force veteran
whose stubborn charm enchanted
and exasperated us during his two
decades on the streets of our city.
Rumor was that he had been drafted
by the Boston Bruins after a stellar
high-school hockey career. On a
frigid and snowy night three days
after Christmas, he was found on
a cement bench two blocks from
Massachusetts General Hospital.

His core body temperature was 78°F. Our team had checked in with him earlier in the evening in the bitter cold on Cambridge Street, and we did our best to urge him to go to Pine Street Inn or to McInnis House, but he insisted he was fine. The cause of death remains uncertain, although he likely suffered a seizure in the hours before he was found so hypothermic. Heroic measures in the emergency room to "warm" him with heated saline given intravenously and through chest tubes placed in the pleural space of both lungs failed to restore a heart rhythm.

The subterranean ceremony was evocative: songs sung to piano, guitar, and trumpet; poems of loss and hope; readings from the Old Testament; tears punctuated by peals of laughter as stories were shared by his many friends and acquaintances. The wide circle of caregivers was a particular surprise to all of us; it included emergency room nurses, social workers, outreach street workers, therapists from the mental health community, and ourselves. This ebullient man had logged legendary numbers of visits to the MGH emergency department, earning a virtually permanent gurney in the hallway. He was known for blowing kisses to nurses, rarely refusing meals, and never failing to offer profound thanks to each person who cared for him. Malcolm was on a first-name basis with the staff of the homeless outreach team of the Department of Mental Health. The nurses at Andrew House lamented the loss of a man who had tried literally hundreds of detoxifications in this dual diagnosis unit, but who had never managed to achieve more than a few weeks of sober time. We couldn't help but share a single sad curiosity: did Malcolm realize how many lives he had touched during his solitary life on the streets, or how many people cared so much about him that they gathered on a frigid wintry day to celebrate his life and memory?

I last saw him on Christmas Eve as I was finishing inpatient rounds at MGH. I got off the elevator on White 9, and he was sitting proudly by the window in the small lobby area, looking off toward the frozen Charles River and eating a turkey dinner that had been brought to him by Denyce Stanton, a nurse who had befriended him during his innumerable admissions. She had seen him downstairs alone in the main hospital lobby and had coaxed him up to the floor for a meal and a flurry of attention by the nurses and the medical team. He was ecstatic and grateful.

"The mashed potatoes are lumpy and no turnips tonight. And this turkey would be succulent with a little Chardonnay!"

His shoes were warming on the radiator, and his swollen feet were a podiatrist's textbook: hammer toes, bunions, stasis dermatitis, old frostbite, onychomycosis, and marked lichenification and pitting typical of immersion foot. The stench was stupefying, and the evening visitors kept a wide berth. I invited him to come to Barbara McInnis House for the holiday, but he graciously declined with an expansive gesture that let me know he had all he needed for now.

Malcolm didn't share much of his past, although he once admitted that he had been married and had lost contact with his two children. No family members have been located since his death, and his hulking body remained unclaimed in the city morgue for the requisite six months before cremation and internment in a paupers' field. We are not even sure of his real name.

The experience of illness and suffering among persons living without homes in urban and rural America is complex and poorly understood. Malcolm's saga is numbingly familiar to physicians, nurses, and other clinicians who witness the lonely, desperate, and painful deaths of homeless men and women in our inner city hospitals and academic medical centers. Death is a constant, albeit erratic, presence on the streets. We know from our own studies in Boston, as well as from studies across the globe, that homeless persons suffer mortality rates that are at least fourfold higher than those of the general population. This is the case in New York City, Philadelphia, San Francisco, and Atlanta, as well as Sydney, London, Toronto, Osaka, and Stockholm.

Rough sleepers are an eclectic group of resolute individuals who embrace a modern brand of rugged American individualism and who eschew the rules and crowds of the shelters. Feisty and complex, stubborn and uncompromising, these persons can alternately exasperate and endear themselves to us. Despite their ubiquitous presence on the urban American landscape, these impoverished individuals' tragic lives remain hidden and obscure. As was Jeremiah preaching to the exiles, rough sleepers are urban nomads who dwell under bridges, in subway tunnels, and down back alleys—modern prophets on the fringes of society who emerge to rant, regale, and condemn a world gone astray.

I once thought of rough sleepers as hearty survivors. In January 2000 our team began following a cohort of 119 people who had been living on the streets of Boston for six consecutive months or more. Most had lived on the streets for five years or longer. Despite an average age of only 45 when our subjects first began this study, a third of these individuals were dead within five years. The leading causes of death were cancer, heart disease, and liver disease. Our hypothesis that these individuals had fallen through the holes in our safety net and had avoided our health care system proved resoundingly wrong. In a scathing rebuke of my own profession, Medicaid reported that these 119 individuals had an aggregate 18,384 emergency room visits in the five years between 1999 and 2003. We are only beginning to understand the ethical and financial costs of our society's neglect of those who live chronically on our streets without access to safe and affordable housing.

The Barbara McInnis House often becomes the venue for the deaths of rough sleepers. Our nurses and doctors tread that fine line between caregiver and family member, as we are often the only "family" for dying homeless persons. Several years ago we diagnosed an undocumented 42-year-old man from Central America with a leiomyosarcoma. A tireless worker at Suffolk Downs, a thoroughbred racetrack just past Logan Airport on the border of East Boston and Revere, this man lived in a stall in one of the barns on the backstretch and sent half of his meager wages to his impoverished family. He was admitted to McInnis House after his initial surgery, and he underwent monthly chemotherapy that left him frail and fatigued. His response to treatment was disappointing, and his medical and nursing care became intense as he weakened. We referred him to a skilled nursing facility for hospice care. This taciturn man tearfully pleaded to stay in the place where he felt safe and accepted. We didn't know how to send him away. Virtually everyone volunteered to take turns sitting with him at night to monitor his pain, help him to the commode, and ease his dread of dying alone. Hospice nurses came to McInnis House to assist with his care and to educate us in end-of-life care. He died peacefully and with minimal pain two months later. The time and intensity of these efforts were exhausting, and they created considerable tension for our beleaguered staff. Yet all were grateful for the opportunity. Perhaps most surprisingly, the fears of our other patients were allayed with the realization that they would not be abandoned at the time of death.

Each death poses unique challenges. Bob Miller, a 50-year-old Vietnam veteran who spent twenty years living in Boston Common, developed head and neck cancer soon after celebrating a year of sobriety. His medical odyssey included a "commando" surgical procedure after he failed to respond to weeks of radiation therapy and two courses of chemotherapy. His mandible and tongue were excised and reconstructed with a bone from his pelvis and a muscle flap from his thigh. When not in the hospital, he was in our respite care program, where he stubbornly managed his own tracheostomy care while still smoking in the courtyard. A deepening depression, explosive outbursts over innocuous comments by other patients, and an escalating dependency on opiates for pain control became contentious and frightening, and he was eventually transferred to a nursing home for the last three months of his life. We would visit him regularly, although we would endure his wrath whenever we missed a day or failed to bring cigarettes or a Dunkin' Donuts large coffee with extra cream and eight sugars. Unable to muster even a nod of thanks from his disfigured face, he left a poem of hope and gratitude in his bedside drawer to be read at his funeral.

The streets can be desperate, lonely, and deadly. Rough sleepers have been exiled to the fringes of our cities—prophets and visionaries gone astray who illuminate the failures of many sectors of our society, including housing, education, health, welfare, labor, and corrections. Choices and options have been limited by the ravages of poverty, illiteracy, mental illness, addictions, cognitive deficits, traumatic brain injuries, and chronic medical illnesses. These cries from the urban desert rattle our foundations.

Zagnut Bars

OCTOBER 2006

Earlier this evening the team on White
11 at MGH called to let me know that
Matthew Diamond had died peacefully.
His friend Daniel Parnell was at his
side. Death is numbingly familiar in
our world, but Matthew was born
two months before me, and somehow
his story and his tender friendship
with Daniel shattered my "concerned
detachment."

Born in hardscrabble Brockton, the home of boxer Rocky Marciano, Matthew had nine siblings and passed inattentively through ten grades. He rarely spoke about his past save for rare oblique comments about working in the shipyards, time in prison, and a broken marriage. His substance-use history was somewhat unusual. An inveterate drinker since his early teens, replete with multiple DUIs, detoxifications, and failed attempts at sobriety, Matthew quit alcohol completely at age 50 and shifted abruptly to heroin. Living for eight years in his car and eventually on the streets, he reminded me of the old and revered jazz musicians whose heroin was a mellow muse that kept the harsher realities of poverty and hopelessness at bay. Matthew was engaging and humorous, occasionally cantankerous, but never violent. Alcohol and hepatitis C (from his needle use) were dual insults to his liver, and over the past several years he progressed inexorably to cirrhosis and end-stage liver disease. And now the final insult was an aggressive liver cancer (hepatocellular carcinoma) that had spread throughout his emaciated body.

My relationship with Matthew began at the Boston Night Center, where he regularly sought refuge during the winter months. The Night Center is a remarkable evening drop-in site designed to attract the street folks who can't tolerate the rules or the crowds of the shelters. Located on the second floor of a city-owned building in Boston's West End, the Night Center is run by Pine Street Inn in space that serves as a Department of Mental Health clubhouse during the day. We have a medical clinic at the Night Center each Wednesday night from 8:30PM until 10PM, after which we join the van for the remainder of the night. The van and the Boston Night Center have been the foundation of our efforts to provide continuity of care to the street folks.

Matthew had the usual skin infections and abscesses that haunt heroin users, and occasionally he would agree to go to McInnis House for care. He won the hearts of everyone there, although he rarely lasted more than a few days before restlessness and yearning propelled him back to the streets and back to heroin. He always left ashamed, grateful for the care, and surprised that we would welcome him back.

In the last year or so, his liver disease left him bloated and fatigued. He came frequently to McInnis House after hospitalizations at MGH for intestinal hemorrhages, pneumonia, and other complications of his cirrhosis.

Matthew befriended Daniel Parnell during long hours sitting on the wall at Park Station. Jill Roncarati, our street team's physician assistant, and Cheryl Kane, our nurse, would see them virtually every day. Daniel was eligible for our housing-first pilot, and after three decades on the streets and months in McInnis House he now has an apartment, owned by Pine Street Inn's innovative Paul Sullivan Housing Trust, in a brownstone on Beacon Street in Brookline.

Quirky and obsessive, Daniel once fell down the steps across from the State House, fractured both of his ankles, then stubbornly walked four blocks to South Station, took the train to Holbrook, and limped through the snow to the emergency room of the local hospital. "I can't stand the hospitals in Boston." During his prolonged stays at Barbara McInnis House, his paranoia necessitated a private room and oodles of attention from nursing and medical staff. He has slowly adjusted to his new home. He sits proudly in the bay window and greets everyone coming in and out of the building. He hasn't wanted a bed as yet, preferring to sleep on the floor wrapped in the government-issue blankets that we gave him each night on the van.

Daniel does not have a substance-use problem and disdains heroin use and heroin addicts. Yet somehow he and Matthew became fast friends. I remember seeing them both at McInnis House last Thanksgiving. Matthew was doing their laundry while Daniel sat lazily in a chair. Matthew whispered to me that he had to do these things because Daniel would never be able to do them himself. Daniel coyly explained that he was always trying to find "chores" for Matthew to do so that he would be distracted from his craving for heroin.

Over these past two weeks, Matthew deteriorated and became markedly jaundiced. His belly was distended, his legs grossly edematous, and his scrotum swollen to the size of a soccer ball. We tried to admit him to MGH on at least two occasions, but he left the emergency room after his initial evaluations. We saw him on Monday and Wednesday evening last week at the Boston Night Center, and he promised to come to our MGH Street Clinic on Thursday morning as usual. When he hadn't appeared by the afternoon, Jill engaged Daniel to go find him and to coax him into the hospital. Later that evening, the emergency room attending doctor called, and we went to see Matthew. Resolute to help his friend, Daniel was sitting in the bay next to Matthew's gurney. Matthew agreed to an admission, although he lingered in the emergency room for almost 36 hours before a bed was available on White 11. Over the ensuing days, Daniel was constantly with him, leaving only when visiting hours ended at 11PM each night. Matthew wept with Daniel's departure each night, afraid that he would die alone. The nurses were initially befuddled by Daniel's appearance and quirky demeanor, but they came to find him a godsend in helping to ease Matthew's anxiety and fear of being alone in the hospital.

Because my father was also a patient in Massachusetts General Hospital this past week, I have had a chance to see Matthew each day. Jill and Jason Sousa, our devoted and phenomenal third-year Harvard Medical student, joined me to visit Matthew on Saturday. We stumbled into a raging argument. Matthew was unsteadily trying to dress and was adamant about heading directly to the streets.

"I'm dying and I need to smoke."

The nurses were willing to bend the rules, but they were too busy at that time to accompany him outside. So I volunteered to be the chaperone, while Jill was summarily dispatched to satisfy Matthew's plea for a Zagnut bar. Neither Jill nor I had ever heard of Zagnut bars, and the wacky name had us wondering if Matthew was hallucinating a bit. Daniel rose to his defense and pointed out that in the 1982 movie *48 Hours*, Nick Nolte took convict Eddie Murphy out to dinner and only offered him a Zagnut bar. First made in 1930, the bar consists of crunchy peanut brittle and a bit of cocoa covered in coconut. With no chocolate coating to melt in the heat, this bar enjoyed a resurgence in popularity as a favorite of troops fighting in Desert Storm in Iraq.

Daniel and I wheeled Matthew down Fruit Street to have what was to be his last cigarette. Matthew savored the first long drag the way I remember dying soldiers in old war films smoking cigarettes after being wounded in the battlefields. He breathed in the cool air as Daniel joked about getting a skateboard for him. Jill showed up with several Zagnut bars she had found in a store along Charles Street, and Matthew howled with delight as he devoured one with eyes closed and head thrown back. He laughed and made us promise not to feel sorry for him.

"I did all this to myself."

Then he pleaded for us to take him to McInnis House, to get rid of the tubes and IVs, and to find his street clothes.

"Why do they make us wear these ridiculous hospital johnnys anyway?"

I admitted the gowns are ridiculous and humiliating. The origin of the term is debated, but I have always been told that the name "johnny" refers to the open back that made it easy for patients to use the john, or toilet.

Matthew was now chilled, and we went back upstairs to White 11. I thought we might have a week or two at that point, but his kidneys stopped working, and his lungs filled with cancer that metastasized from his liver. On Sunday we had the "talk," as he called it. He was alert and vigilant, and he politely declined dialysis and other interventions that might give him a little more time. "No more poking. It's time to die." He firmly declared that we should not bother his family.

On Monday night we stopped by his room with the crew from the Pine Street Inn van, and Matthew was thrilled to see familiar folks. His eyes were vivid yellow, and his body swollen and disfigured. The next morning Sarah Ciambrone and Dr. Monica Bharel and the staff at McInnis House graciously agreed to accept Matthew for end-of-life care, although no beds would be available until the next day. But time was not his, and Matthew gradually slipped into a coma on Tuesday and died peacefully at 6PM.

Daniel was with him throughout his hospitalization, and Matthew died holding Daniel's hand. Some things we cannot predict or understand, only accept and cherish. Matthew was a hardened steel worker and heroin addict afraid of dying alone, and Daniel a solitary and complex loner who reviles drugs and alcohol. In the long litany of deaths on the streets, the end of Matthew's arduous journey had a sweet and rare tenderness.

Resilience

APRIL 2008

I first met Susan Valencia during a
Nor'easter several years ago. Freezing
and trembling in an encampment along
the railroad tracks near Andrew Square
in South Boston, she stared blankly
at her purple and black toes in the
flickering light cast by the flames of a
pair of Sternos. After much cajoling she
came into the van and agreed to let us
take her to the emergency room.

The triage nurse at Boston Medical Center graciously allowed us to leapfrog the red tape of registration and ushered us directly to a gurney in the hallway on the acute-trauma side of the emergency department. Susan was rapidly evaluated and admitted for hypothermia and frostbite, worrisome harbingers of the complications that would soon beset her and overwhelm us.

Susan defied the odds and lost only two toes, and within a few months she was back with her boyfriend Jose in the encampment. She was the sole woman among several raucous but hard-working homeless men from Central and South America. Many memories from that time emerge: Susan, part Native American, didn't speak a word of Spanish, and her boyfriend couldn't speak English; only 23, Susan hid her past, quietly read a book a day in the hospital, and was void of any self-pity; Susan's life was precarious under her bridge, an infamous place where Mario from El Salvador had been beaten to death with a baseball bat by a local gang of teenagers that previous summer. In the years after that first night's trip to the ED, we saw Susan frequently on the van. She was polite and welcoming, but beyond accepting our soup, sandwiches, and blankets, she was never interested in our offers to help.

During a blizzard in the midst of another bitter cold spell two winters ago, we found Susan alone along the railroad tracks with severe hypothermia and frostbite of her toes. Gangrene complicated her recovery at Brigham and Women's Hospital, and she required an amputation of her left leg below the knee. Her stoicism was unsettling, and I was struck by her calm demeanor and flat affect in the face of her life-threatening ordeal. The psychiatrist shared my concerns but thought Susan was competent and able to make her own decisions. Cooperative and endearing, she still read a book each day, and her boyfriend remained devoted and visited often. After several weeks in the hospital and a prolonged stint at McInnis House to learn to use her new prosthesis, Susan returned again to the streets, declining our fervent offers of shelter, housing, or programs.

Susan's relationships with Jose and heroin grew sinewy. Last spring she had developed a high fever and had difficulty breathing. At Boston Medical Center she was found to be severely ill with heart failure caused by an infection of one of her heart valves, a condition known as bacterial endocarditis. The bacteria had entered her system when she injected heroin, and the treatment required two months of intravenous (IV) antibiotics. During the second week of her admission, Susan was found unconscious and not breathing. She revived during the "code blue," although the respiratory arrest had been caused by an accidental overdose of heroin that her boyfriend had helped her inject directly into her IV catheter. Her health rapidly deteriorated as aggressive new types of bacteria infected the heart valve, and she required additional broad-spectrum antibiotics. Susan agreed to the treatment plan of two more months of IV antibiotics as well as methadone to treat her heroin dependence. After a month, she was transferred to McInnis House for the completion of her antibiotics and the continuation of her cardiac care.

Several dramas unfolded during her stay at McInnis House. She mustered the courage to break from her abusive relationship with Jose, despite his daily visits. Almost immediately, she was smitten by Alberto, a fellow patient at BMH, who had recently been released from a prolonged incarceration, and who boisterously vowed to be her protector. Despite the gentle and consistent voicing of our fears to Susan, she was resolute and not to be deterred or swayed. The amazing McInnis House staff spent many hours trying to find a suitable placement for Susan. Much to our chagrin, Susan left McInnis House just before Christmas with Alberto, who promised to take her to a local hotel for the holidays.

Commitments

JULY 2008

This morning will be bittersweet. Our McInnis House patients will be moving to the renovated Mallory Institute of Pathology, and the excitement has been as palpable as the trepidation. We are eager to witness the reactions of our patients as they enter the Cary W. Akins Pavilion and finally see the new Jean Yawkey Place. Most will be overwhelmed by the beauty and dignity of the surroundings and will have a hard time accepting that this is meant for them.

An abiding sadness lingers as we close the doors of our beloved Barbara McInnis House on the border between Roxbury and Jamaica
Plain, and vivid memories of that earlier move percolate through my
consciousness. Just over fifteen years ago, we took a plunge into a
vast unknown. We purchased Stadium Manor on Walnut Avenue,
white-washed the walls, and moved our 25-bed "medical respite unit"
from a corner of the Lemuel Shattuck Shelter to this former nursing home. Twenty-five bewildered patients climbed into our vans,
journeyed across Franklin Park to our new home, and were served
a buffet lunch in the lobby. We were undoubtedly the proudest folks
in all of Boston.

Until that moment, we had been "guests" in every place we
worked—shelters, soup kitchens, motels, and hospitals. An exhaustive four-year search for a building and for sustainable funding for
our respite-care services had finally come to an end. Our budget and
our staff tripled virtually overnight. Just to keep us from celebrating
too much, we now had responsibility for a host of new 24/7 challenges, including meals, laundry, roof leaks, and three shifts of staff. The
change was radical, but we shared a collective sense that this journey
through uncharted territory was worth the risk. With great devotion
from our BHCHP staff, patients, and friends, the cinderblock building on that huge granite slab near Eggleston Square soon became a
warm and loving testament to the unique spirit and feisty resilience
of Barbara McInnis. Closing those doors will hurt in the very best
of ways.

During our street-team meeting this week, we grappled with the
ethical and moral implications of civil commitments for folks we believe are too vulnerable to be staying on the streets. This dilemma
over civil liberties has haunted us for years without clear resolution,
so forgive any ambivalence. Our arsenal of street tools includes two
means of involuntary commitment for individuals whom we feel are
in "imminent" danger of harming themselves or others. Section 12 is
for those whose judgment is compromised by mental illness, and the
process starts with the treatment system, not the courtroom. When

we find an individual who is flagrantly psychotic and in peril on the streets or in the shelters, we sign a Section 12 form and call 911. The individual is then taken to the nearest emergency room for a full psychiatric evaluation within 48 hours, after which a determination about mandatory hospitalization is made. We have had mixed success with this process, although the outcomes have often been good.

When an individual is in danger with impaired judgment due to alcohol or drugs, we have only Section 35 to invoke. This starts with the courtroom. We have judiciously utilized this rather blunt tool in the past, as our outcomes to date have been dismal. The process requires the doctor (or family member, policeman, or clergyman) to physically appear in court and to petition the judge for a Section 35 by offering evidence of imminent danger necessitating a commitment. If the judge agrees, a 24-hour warrant is issued for the apprehension of the individual. The police need to know where to find the person, and thus it is critical that we know the whereabouts of the patient on the day we make such an appeal to the court. The police then arrest and transport the individual to the court, where a lawyer is assigned to the case. The doctor must then testify in court before the judge and the patient with the lawyer. This jeopardizes our relationship with the patient, who sits in the court room in handcuffs while we articulate our concerns. If the court agrees with us, then the men are sent to the Massachusetts Correctional Institution at Bridgewater (MCIB), and the women are sent to either Framingham Prison or one of several recovery programs sanctioned by the state. The usual length of time is 30 days. The process is bruising, and we have rarely had anyone maintain periods of sobriety once released.

Several years ago I languished for hours in the West Roxbury Courthouse in an attempt to commit Jim Danforth, a 43-year-old man who had lived for a decade on the streets, to MCIB under Section 35. We had grown increasingly fearful for his safety in the previous six months, as daily alcohol and Listerine had rendered him helpless on the sidewalks of Downtown Crossing, and a series of worsening head injuries led to admissions to the ICUs of Beth Is-

rael Deaconess Medical Center, New England Medical Center, and
Massachusetts General Hospital. He fractured his neck, had at least
two serious hemorrhages into his brain tissue necessitating bore holes
through the skull for drainage, and had a large subdural hematoma, a
bruise between his brain and skull that required surgical evacuation.
He repeatedly left the hospital and returned to Downtown Crossing,
where he neglected the most basic skills of living. One hot summer
night the EMTs brought him unconscious to the emergency room at
Massachusetts General Hospital. He was covered in urine and feces
and infested with so many maggots that even the seasoned nurses
were aghast. The usual treatments didn't work, and his groin and rec-
tum had to be packed with ground beef to attract the maggots away
from his body, a strategy I had seen used only once before.

After ten days in the hospital, he was found unable to make
sound judgments about his medical care, but he somehow managed
to abscond to the streets yet again. Within two days he was brought
to Beth Israel Deaconess Medical Center with further head trauma
and another hemorrhage into his brain. That compelled us to seek
the Section 35, which was overseen with great care and tenderness by
Judge Robert Rufo at the West Roxbury Court. Our concern about
Jim's ultimate safety led us on yet another journey to the infamous
Titicut Road in Bridgewater last Friday. To our chagrin, Jim was still
in a wheelchair (after 24 days) and did not recognize or remember
us. He was vague about his whereabouts, and he could not remember
any of the many colorful episodes that we had shared together over
the years. He had not participated in any of the treatment available,
and he said that he wanted to return to the streets and have a drink.
I was not surprised, as the extent of his traumatic brain injury and
the effects of his alcoholism were undoubtedly severe. We pointed
out his dramatic mental-status change and the dire need for an evaluation, but the MCIB staff felt that their hands were tied and that
they would have to release him when the court-mandated 30 days
had elapsed.

On Wednesday of this week, we returned to the courthouse

and worked feverishly with the clinic staff to find an alternative to releasing him to the streets. The judge also felt limited in his options because Jim's court-appointed lawyer did not find him impaired, and we did not possess enough formal neurological data to prove our case. The dilemma is familiar and infuriating. A period of sobriety is required to obtain valid neuro-psychiatric testing to assess competency, but such testing is not available at the corrections system at Bridgewater, where Jim would have been sober for a month. Once released, he would be drinking again, so meeting the burden of proof required by the courts would be next-to-impossible. We lost our plea, and he was released to the streets on the day he completed his 30 days.

These stories rarely turn out as expected. Jim didn't go back to his favorite spot at Downtown Crossing, and he didn't drink when he was released. Rather, he returned to the West Roxbury Courthouse, wandered the grounds aimlessly, and eventually fell asleep on the marble steps of the building that night. The next morning he was found by the court psychologist as he arrived at work. Jim was confused and did not know where he was, but we were able to get him to agree to go to McInnis House. He could not remember me when I saw him there, and he had no recollection of where he had been for the past several months. He stared vacuously at all of the people who had cared for him for so long. We devoted months to obtaining a guardian for him, and Jim was placed in a nursing home just outside Boston, where he has been quiet and content for the past five years.

Most recently, Malcolm Dilworth and Larry Walters have emerged as the most frequent visitors at MGH's emergency department. Concerned clinicians at the hospital decided that an involuntary commitment was warranted for the two men's safety and welfare, and the clinicians worked with us to "Section 35" each of them directly from the hospital. We appealed to the judge at Boston Municipal Court, who issued the required warrants, and our two patients were apprehended from the hospital and committed to Bridgewater for 30 days.

Suzanne Armstrong, the wonderful nurse practitioner at McInnis House who has now joined our street team, and Jill Roncarati, our team's physician assistant for many years, worked closely with the staff at MCIB to orchestrate a practical plan for Malcolm Dilworth. When Malcolm was apprehended for the Section 35, an outstanding warrant was uncovered, and the judge mandated that Malcolm return directly to court upon his release from MCIB. Jill and Jessica Lanney, our Princeton summer intern, went to Boston Municipal Court on the morning of Malcolm's release to meet with the judge and the court psychologist. The old warrant was dismissed as long as Malcolm would agree to be admitted directly to McInnis House for continued care. Rather than angry, he felt relieved and grateful, kissing Jill's hand as she escorted him to the cab to go to McInnis House. Reflecting on his run of alcohol in the weeks before his Section 35, Malcolm said, "I was drinking to die." The coordination and continuity of his care was remarkable, from MCIB to court to McInnis House, and he has now been with us for almost a week and expresses a keen desire to remain sober.

Larry Walters had a more familiar and discouraging course. Unlike Malcolm, he had no outstanding warrants, and MCIB had no choice but to release him after the mandated 30 days. He refused all offers of transitional programs and halfway houses. On July 3, the day of his release, he returned to the streets of Boston and was back in the MGH emergency department within six hours. He has been in the ED each day for the past week, and the cycle has resumed with exuberance. This experience has also eroded much of the trust that we had worked so hard to build with Larry, and he is bitterly angry that we "sent him to jail."

We are bereft of creative and effective treatment options for chronically homeless persons with severe and chronic alcoholism and drug abuse. While most have had multiple detox admissions, the lack of available and timely recovery-home beds and halfway-house beds has rendered the five-day detox programs revolving doors. Even if timely treatment beds were available, most of our chronic street folks have long since failed the best treatment modalities we have, including Alcoholics Anonymous (AA), cognitive behavioral therapy (CBT), and motivational interviewing. As we venture further into the world of housing those who have experienced chronic homelessness, substance-abuse treatment has emerged as one of our most vexing challenges.

Nectar and Nemesis

DECEMBER 2009

I've been burning the proverbial midnight oil over the past two weeks on Bigelow 11 at Massachusetts General Hospital. This annual immersion into daily life on the inpatient medical service has been a wonderful, albeit exhausting, way to keep up-to-date with dizzying changes, occurring with accelerating frequency and complexity, in medicine and patient care.

My contribution to the long-suffering team of interns and residents is a view from the street accompanied by an emphasis on pragmatic treatment plans that acknowledge the diverse living situations of the patients admitted to MGH. The two perspectives collide often, and we have learned much from each other.

The most poignant and evocative moment of this month came the day after Thanksgiving. We received our first gift in our 25-year history from a grateful patient: $11,000.74 from the estate of David Colton. The check was accompanied by a touching note from Jennifer Foxwell, his HomeStart worker, who serves as the representative payee for our folks placed in low-threshold housing, and with whom I worked for years when she drove the Pine Street Inn van. Several weeks before he was found dead in his Quincy apartment, David had willed his entire "estate" to our street team and to the Barbara McInnis House. We had cared for him for many years on the streets, in the hospital, in respite care, and in housing. He always referred to us as his "family" and listed us as next-of-kin in all of his diverse medical records and housing applications. As in many families, our relationship with David was never easy.

David lived on the streets intermittently for decades. I first met him in the Pine Street Inn Clinic in the late 1990s. He told me he had been living with his "best friend," who had recently died and had left David homeless. I grew to know him mostly through the van, in which we would visit him in his cardboard box placed under a loading dock at the Wise potato chip factory in South Boston. A jovial drinker, he would burst into his special rendition of the theme song to *Gilligan's Island*, singing (badly) all of the words and then collapsing with laughter on his knees. He remembered each episode, and I'm sure he escaped into distant memories that he never shared during the years we cared for him. He hailed from New Jersey, mentioned a divorce, but never offered the name of a town or any family members. Some friends on the street told us he had grown up in an orphanage.

He suffered the usual ravages of life on the streets, with multiple blows to his head from falls and fights, several epidural hemorrhages, fractures of his ribs and ankles, and frostbite of his toes. Years of smoking had eroded his lungs and left him with bullous emphysema, while his drinking left him with difficulty swallowing and a pre-cancerous condition called Barrett's esophagus. Demons pursued him relentlessly, resulting in admissions to hospitals and mental health centers for suicidal ideation and thoughts of self-loathing and worthlessness. Alcohol was both nectar and nemesis, and over the years we admitted him to innumerable detoxification units and post-detoxification programs as he struggled heroically to string together days and weeks of sobriety.

David came many times to the old Barbara McInnis House on Walnut Avenue, where he had rapidly become a darling of the nurses and the aides. He was polite, respectful, grateful, fun. All of his recent periods of sobriety began with admissions to McInnis House. In the summer of 2006, he was admitted from the streets disheveled and distraught, and he stayed six months before going to the Salvation Army in Cambridge and then into Paul Sullivan Housing, where he had a room in a congregate setting on Half Moon Street in Dorchester. The tenancy was rocky, but he managed almost a year before he was evicted for drinking and poor hygiene. He then returned to the streets of South Boston. When he was admitted to McInnis House after this failed attempt at housing, he had changed significantly. The infectious laughter dissolved in vitriol and malcontent. He argued with staff and patients, criticized his care, and moaned that "no one was helping me." In the summer of 2008, he was placed in a one-bedroom apartment on the fourth floor of a building in Quincy through our housing-first pilot program with HomeStart, a local housing organization dedicated to finding just and equitable housing for poor and homeless populations. The pilot was a joint "housing first" venture of BHCHP and HomeStart with the Massachusetts Behavioral Health Partnership. The goal was to house the most chronic street folks and to orchestrate an array of health and supportive services in their new homes. Medicaid paid for the services of the housing worker. This new and exciting effort underscored the belief that stable housing is likely to improve health and reduce health care costs in emergency rooms and hospitals. The people housed through this program had been living chronically on the streets since at least 2000, and David was on the list.

Despite months of sobriety in McInnis House, he began drinking immediately in his new home, and he pushed the limits of his landlord's tolerance despite our constant intercession. He neglected his personal hygiene, used a bucket in the living room as his toilet, set fires while cooking, stumbled and fell repeatedly on the stairs. The police and the EMTs came to know him by first name as he began a series of admissions to Quincy Medical Center that left everyone deeply concerned for his welfare. He was always deemed competent to make his own decisions, despite having presented covered in urine and feces, with a dangerously low sodium level and a rare condition called central pontine myelinolysis. As he said at the time: "I haven't eaten anything for weeks. All I can do is drink."

His landlord agreed to let him move to an apartment on the first floor of his building rather than to evict him. His room on the fourth floor was beyond filthy and required exterminators and professional cleaners before repainting. The rugs and the furniture had to be thrown into the trash. So we moved him to his third apartment, where he did well for a week before relapsing. He avoided us assiduously, despite many knocks on his door.

On August 4 of this past summer, his landlord found him dead in his room. The cause of his death remains unknown, as the Medical Examiner found no clear medical problem, other than alcoholism, to account for his death at the age of 49. We did not know that he had met a few weeks before with Jennifer to discuss his will, leaving us to wonder if the series of failures had taken a toll, quelling his laughter and extinguishing his resolve to fight his disease. Sarah Ciambrone, longtime director of McInnis House, noted that David struggled to do the right thing but was always thwarted.

I called the Medical Examiner this week to see if David was still in the morgue. No family members were located, and he is now buried in a paupers' field somewhere in Massachusetts. We want to honor his memory and to celebrate the extraordinary gifts he gave to those of us privileged to care for him...not to mention the singular and historic monetary gift to BHCHP.

Remembering 9/11/2001

SEPTEMBER 2011

Ten years ago, on the afternoon of the World Trade Center attacks, Cheryl Kane and Sharon Morrison, our wise and restless street-team nurses, sallied over to my desk and prodded me out of my torpor. Some homeless folks had called from Andrew Square, and we needed to get back to work. During our monthly Board of Directors meeting that morning in Steve Tringale's office next to Boston City Hall, Peter Meade got a call alerting us to a report that a small plane had allegedly hit the North Tower of the World Trade Center.

Looking across the harbor from our meeting room on the 29th floor, we soon realized that the usual buzz of activity had ceased and that no planes were landing or taking off at Logan Airport. Soon thereafter we were caught in the mass evacuation of all buildings in downtown Boston. Exiting the Post Office Square underground garage and driving the six blocks across town to our offices adjacent to Boston Medical Center took almost three hours, underscoring the helplessness and paralysis that gripped us all that morning. I listened in disbelief to NPR and tried to visualize the crumbling of those massive Twin Towers.

At 2PM, I drove Cheryl and Sharon through our eerily deserted city to an abandoned lot near Andrew Square. The lot was adjacent to a truck and bus junkyard and was separated from the busy Southeast Expressway by abandoned railroad tracks. Three days earlier Peter Simpson's rigid body, sallow and bloated by cirrhosis, had been found sitting upright against a stone wall in this same clearing. Kate Travis and Robert Hollins now sat with legs extended in tattered and bent beach chairs in the overgrown field. They gesticulated wildly and hurled insults at each other. Bobby Cox paced at a comfortable distance, cursing and vowing to fight America's cowardly enemies hiding across the globe. Kate's face was bruised and battered, her skirt short and torn. Robert's salty tongue and acerbic wit seemed incongruous with a body rendered pale and feeble by the ravages of alcohol and long-ignored diabetes. We sat and commiserated about the morning's events for some time before they would talk about themselves. After taking vital signs and performing cursory physical exams in the field, we coaxed Kate and Robert into a cab and sent them to McInnis House for safety and care.

We then headed downtown and found Joe Chiampa on the waterfront near the Aquarium. Resolutely proud of his country, Joe had tears of helpless rage clouding his reddened eyes and streaming along furrows deepened by sundrenched years fishing in the Georges Bank. Joe slept between the parallel rows of Jersey barriers that divided Atlantic Avenue throughout the long years of Boston's massive

Big Dig. A veritable legend on Boston's waterfront for 30 years, Joe's characteristic single-shoulder shrug, piercing blue eyes, scabrous wit, and steely streak of independence were enveloped by an endearing charm, not to mention the once-bright-yellow parka which doubled magnificently as a beacon whenever we went to find him along Atlantic Avenue. He was fiercely protective of that jacket, given to him by Cheryl on Christmas Day of 2000. Cheryl recalls that he initially looked askance at the jacket that had belonged to her husband Jim, and Joe questioned why Jim had rejected it. She explained that Jim had recently died of a brain tumor, but she knew that he would be honored to have Joe wear his favorite parka. Joe then put his arm around Cheryl and did his best to comfort her. He wore that jacket with great pride.

Joe was a raconteur who regaled us with stories, real and imaginary: owning a fleet of fishing boats at Commonwealth Pier, playing halfback at Michigan, wild celebrations of his birthday on Pearl Harbor Day. He weathered bitterly cold nights and blistering summer heat, and he even survived a near-drowning and massive heart attack when he was assaulted and thrown into Boston Harbor two years ago. Interestingly, he was rescued by Arthur Nardi, another rough sleeper, who selflessly dove into the frigid waters and steadfastly refused recognition or credit.

"Any friend would have done the same thing."

Roy Morrison, a wise advocate who has worked with Pine Street Inn for years, remarked that half of downtown Boston was "co-dependent" on Joe. A coterie of devoted Big Dig workers, Harbor Tower residents, and business folks from the Aquarium to the Boston Harbor Hotel regularly offered clothing, food, and even invitations to holiday dinners at their homes. Our street team checked on him most days, and the overnight van stopped on Atlantic Street each night to ensure he had food and a blanket. Try as we might to bring him in, Joe's manifold objections to the rules and crowds of shelters narrowed his options, although he would periodically seek warmth for a few hours at the Boston Night Center, a drop-in center designed to serve those who preferred living on the streets to staying in shelters. When he was too sick and feeble, he would acquiesce to an admission to McInnis House, where he was comfortable with the nurses and doctors. The wanderlust always returned as his health improved. Afraid of disappointing us or appearing ungrateful, he would quietly abscond through the back door and wend his way back to Atlantic Avenue.

Farther along the wharf we found a sullen trio of stalwarts in Columbus Park on the edge of the North End. The usual banter and bravado were missing, along with the dancing and posturing. The talk somberly focused on the deaths of so many innocent persons. Mary Anne Norbury and Arthur Nardi, Joe's rescuer from Boston Harbor, were inseparable on the streets, but they agreed to go to Andrew House, a public detoxification program on Boston's Long Island. With much pleading and reluctant promises of cigarettes, we convinced Sergio Zermatti to return to Massachusetts General Hospital. We had admitted him several days previously for bleeding from esophageal varices, a complication of his end-stage liver disease. He fled the hospital in a fit of rage after watching the Twin Towers collapse, and I was much relieved that he was willing to return to the hospital.

September 11, 2001, changed life on the streets for a brief but poignant time. The capricious terror of that day captivated and unsettled the lives of the most disenfranchised. The *New York Times* later reported that admissions to shelters for victims of domestic violence dropped precipitously after 9/11, with many shelters across the country closing for a short time. Old Glory appeared on shopping carts, wheelchairs, and cardboard hovels under bridges. Patriotism trumped hopelessness, ancient grudges were buried, and our poorest citizens were fully embraced by a frightened, humbled, and deeply wounded America. But as Indian summer waned, life on the streets faded to normal. Access to public buildings and amenities was curtailed by the new security measures and the requirement of a photo ID. That brief glimpse of a shared patriotism and a new social contract was soon shuttered by a brutal economy that shredded the state budget and widened the gap between rich and poor.

Kate and Robert stayed for a couple of weeks at McInnis House before heading back to alcohol and South Boston. When the weather was warm enough, they would sleep by the L Street bathhouses or in the middle of the ball field on Day Boulevard. On cold days they would ride the Red Line from Ashmont to Cambridge and sleep under the platform in the Andrew Square station. Kate was found frozen to death later that winter. Bobby continued to struggle with heroin and alcohol, but he later found sobriety and began classes at UMass Boston. He is now thriving and working as an addictions counselor.

Joe lived only a few more months. The first snow came in early November, when Joe seemed exhausted and sad about the upcoming holiday season. We found him drunk and passed out on the sidewalk near the Aquarium one cold night, and we orchestrated an admission to the geriatric neuro-psychiatry unit at the Lemuel Shattuck Hospital. Confused and combative during the first days of alcohol withdrawal, he soon cleared, and we had an opportunity to thoroughly evaluate his medical and mental health status. He sailed through the MRIs, EKGs, and blood tests; to our amazement, he aced the memory and competency examinations. No holds were barred as he read me the riot act and expressed his disgust with us when we visited. Suspending the usual formalities, he stormed out after two weeks, resolutely refusing to abdicate his cherished role on the waterfront.

I saw him around midnight a few days after Thanksgiving. Huddled under army-issue blankets between the Jersey barriers, he took a deep drag on his cigarette and wistfully described the stuffed artichokes and mushrooms his friend Susan had cooked for Thanksgiving dinner. His eyes welled with tears as he reminisced about his beloved grandmother and his favorite aunt Lily, and he confessed how he missed his Italian family. On Pearl Harbor Day, he was jovial when we stopped by the Aquarium to celebrate his birthday. A doctor in the emergency room at Boston Medical Center paged me early the next morning to tell me that Joe had been crushed to death when a BMW SUV lost control and rolled over the Jersey barrier on Atlantic Avenue. Several vertebrae in his neck were shattered. A discrepancy in his date of birth kept his body at the morgue for two weeks, but he was finally given to his family.

At the wake in his hometown of Mansfield, we shared laughter and tears with the loving and long-suffering family whom he had described with such affection, and who had tried so often to bring him home. On the Friday of Christmas week we sat among the standing-room-only throng of family and friends at his memorial service at St. Mary's Church, where he had been baptized. After the funeral we went to the family home to celebrate his life. The pictures of a little blond boy shrugging with one shoulder at the camera and of the movie-star handsome high school graduate transfixed us. The stories flowed, ribald and raucous, tender and tragic. Amidst the laughter and tears, we were left to ponder the mystery of what keeps us apart.

His beloved aunt Lily told us that Joe's mother had abandoned him, and Joe spent much time with his grandmother and aunt. Joe's father had a fishing business in Falmouth, and Joe began fishing when he was a very young child, learning a trade in which he would later excel. Joe's father eventually remarried, but his new wife rejected Joe and blamed him for the unhappiness in the marriage. Aunt Lily says Joe never played football for Michigan. He married twice but each time abandoned his own family. He had two children, but no one in Joe's family knows of their whereabouts. During his 30 years on the streets of Boston, he would occasionally come to Mansfield to stay with Lily, and he always brought flowers: "He would stay as long as he could, but one day would go to the store to buy cigarettes and not come back for years. He had a terrible, terrible disease." His grandmother, aunts, and cousins spent a lifetime trying to embrace him, but his wounds were just not the healing kind.

Mary Anne and Arthur returned to the North End, although Arthur suffered from loss of oxygen to his brain during an overdose of heroin and a cocktail of sedatives. He required years of 24-hour care in a nursing home in Jamaica Plain. We visited him regularly even though he couldn't remember who we were. He succumbed to an overwhelming pneumonia in 2009. Sergio left the hospital again, against medical advice, and overdosed on the sidewalk near Kingston House a few weeks later. He cut a Fentanyl patch into small pieces, boiled the pieces in water, and died after drinking the potent opioid broth.

A Modernist's Creed

JULY 2013

Sometimes clinic visits are a deft duel between the literary and the mundane. One of the masters of this art is a former teacher with obsessive-compulsive disorder whom I met during his five years on the streets of Boston. He has spent the past several years in a rented room in Dorchester, and he religiously graces our Thursday Street Clinic at MGH as we manage his chronic and smoldering leukemia as well as atrial fibrillation, a heart arrhythmia for which he takes a daily blood thinner.

Our visits are usually friendly jousts in which the physical signs and symptoms I seek are carefully hidden within majestic literary soliloquies offered by this remarkable septuagenarian. I've tried to capture the essence of a visit near the end of April, when our patients and our staff were traumatized by the Marathon bombings and devastated by the tragic and untimely death of our team's beloved nurse, Stephanie Joy Barker.

"I've been thinking over your vocation because I'm part of your patient group and a regular member of the motley crew in the waiting room downstairs each week. Surely one of the advantages of having as your patients people who are homeless and living on the streets is that they *know* they are in trouble. I could not possibly do what you do because I'm inclined to tell people to shape up. Many are their own worst enemies but one surely can't tell them that. Medicine predates science, and truthfully science didn't make all that much difference. Human beings are human beings. I've been fine since we last met. No blotches have broken out. I'll spare you the remainder of my sermon on homelessness and human nature.

"The bombings at the Boston Marathon last week didn't affect me that much. I was in the cathedral attending a book group. We are reading Willa Cather's *Death Comes for the Archbishop,* a remarkable story of the Southwest that begins with the victorious United States acquiring New Mexico after the Mexican War in 1851. The Vatican posthaste commissioned a new bishop and his assistant to the distant and vast territory. Both of these extraordinary literary characters, as well as others in this novel, are based upon memoirs of real people that had deeply moved Ms. Cather. She was a devout Episcopalian but the fact that her characters were Roman Catholic didn't bother her in the least."

He rummaged through his tote bag and produced a tattered copy of the novel with detailed notes along the margins of every page. His praise for the author was eloquent, punctuated by a rejoinder that I must read *My Antonia* and *Alexander's Bridge.* He went to offer me his own copy, but he stopped when he realized he hadn't yet transcribed his notations.

"Sorry, I put everything I read under a microscope and add my notations to my commonplace book. Ms. Cather is renowned for converting the mundane into a riveting story. The ability to see the remarkable in the seemingly ordinary is the modernist's creed. Authors should be leveling up and not leveling down."

I asked what he meant by that, and he explained that rather than telling stories of grand and glorious things done by people of exalted station, authors should seek meaning in the commonplace and in the ordinary lives we all lead. He pointed out that Cather was a master of narrative who made a clear distinction between story and narrative.

"We are all equidistant from eternity. Read Sartre's *Nausea*...it's funny as the dickens. The narrator is a Catholic who has an epistemological crisis right in the beginning."

At last he was now on my terrain, and I shared my memory of a line in *Nausea* in which the somber narrator is sitting at a bar staring down into his "puddle of beer pressed together by glass." Ouch.

"Friday was the day of sheltering in place. The city was in lockdown but I couldn't sit at home with nothing to do. I ventured out and managed to get this excellent haircut and to balance my checkbook. I was able to walk without fatigue or shortness of breath. No palpitations, and—since Suzanne always inquires—no paroxysmal nocturnal dyspnea!"

After carefully enunciating each of those words, he said it was a jaw-breaker and collapsed in peals of laughter.

"Nineteen-year-old Gavrilo Princip tossed the bomb that killed Archduke Franz Ferdinand of Austria in June of 1914, igniting World War I. He was judged insane and never found guilty of murder, as the Austrians simply could not face the possibility that a person in his right mind would do such an atrocious thing. And now we are facing a similar situation in Boston with this unspeakably heinous act by these two brothers, one of whom is also nineteen. I can't believe that any religious cause could be advanced by such an act. Why should I? While I was in the lab this morning waiting for my weekly vampire stick to check my warfarin levels, I saw their mother on the TV, a very nice looking woman in the traditional head scarf of her people telling what I guess is her side, or maybe her sons' side, of the story. This is dismaying, everything is so complicated and everything has aspects and perspectives and facets and subtleties.

"Willa Cather should come back. This is really shocking. We delude ourselves. A modernist theme is that stories are delusory. Even as a college student I read *Aspects of the Novel* by E.M. Forster, a classic modernist text in which he pooh-poohs the novel and attacks the idea of plot. Have you ever been taught about plot, character, and setting? Well, my friend, there went plot...Pow! Character and setting are next. All we have left are commonplace books and I take time to write in mine each day. I am at last a man of my times.

"I'm with Pascal. I spent a year reading the *Penses*—in translation, mind you. I decided to approach it as a lawyer's brief, assuming these were the notes for a projected defense of the Christian religion. In the course of doing this I realized I was mistaken and things are much better Pascal's way. His way forces the reader to do the thinking. If you think it out for yourself, you are more likely to be convinced. It's also a dare in a sense. He sees the human condition as bleak. His famous similitude is the following: picture for yourself a prison in which day by day some small portion of the inmates are led forth to die—no individual prisoner knows on which particular day he will be called. This is indeed an image of the human condition. I've taken courses in probability theory, which Pascal helped invent, and the expected duration of life for a randomly chosen adult in Pascal's day was about ten years. So one has a decade to shape up and live fully, although in truth tomorrow could be the appointed day of death. So what are the implications? Live life fully in each moment and the mundane is sacred. But people are sad cases and our judgment of ourselves and one another is pathologically bad. We continue to live each day as if we have the whole ten years ahead of us. This book taught me a lot, especially since I naively thought it was just an attempt to convince me that Jesus is my Lord and Savior.

"I'm fine but still in atrial fibrillation. My weight is 154.8 pounds.

The lighter I am the longer it takes for me to have a sense of exertion around the heart. I am trying to keep my weight down without the Lasix, which makes me urinate a half dozen times per night. My landlady and her live-in boyfriend have decided not to bother me anymore and have been nice as pie. I'm waiting for my dossier to rise in the hopper at the two places I have applied for housing, although without looking forward to moving because it's going to be a hell of an ordeal. Putting my books back in boxes is intimidating. Many of the traditional crepitudes of age have so far passed me by...no Parkinsonism, I'm still as deft as I've always been, and no mental decline that I notice. The only thing that's gone is my hearing, and of course this heart condition and the blood dyscrasia lurking in the background. I'm glad you spotted that back in 2006. Feel free to examine me now."

I seized the opportunity to do a focused examination. Everything was normal save for the irregular heart rate. I congratulated him for keeping his mind and his body so active at his age.

"Was it not Aristotle who said that education is the best preparation for old age? Was he right! Most of us sit in front of a TV and quietly waste away. Outside of Scripture, I see this as the most devastating prophecy of the demise of contemporary America. Time to go now. See you when I see you."

The Shoulders of Giants

NOVEMBER 2014

Tom Bennett and his partner Rusty came to my home for a farewell dinner in late 1995. Both were dying of AIDS. Frail and blinded by cytomegalovirus, Tom depended upon Rusty to guide him through each day. Rusty, while still physically robust, had lost all short-term memory to HIV dementia and relied on Tom's lightning-quick mind to negotiate the daily challenges of their life together. Tom's brain and Rusty's body allowed these two magnificent men to function as one.

Tom was a raconteur, irascible and irreverent, and the dinner conversation was lively and full of laughter. Rusty was warm, distant, and content. I have rarely witnessed such joy, resilience, and love in the face of such tragedy.

Tom began working with us when he was a senior resident in medicine at Boston City Hospital in 1987. He elected to do his weekly outpatient clinic with me at Pine Street Inn, and the nurses were awed by his kindness, humor, and ease with homeless persons. He dressed sharply, often in fine Armani suits he would find on sale in Filene's Basement. As Barbara McInnis noted, Tom was "very easy on the eyes."

Tom was a godsend to me and to Robin Avery, who was our only other doctor at that time. She joined us for a year between completing her residency and beginning a fellowship in infectious diseases at Massachusetts General Hospital, and she was truly my salvation in those early days. Robin's energy and clinical skills were extraordinary, and her interest in HIV/AIDS helped us create innovative services for homeless persons within the remarkable and multi-specialty Immunodeficiency Clinic at Boston City Hospital. Robin radiated joy and was beloved by all. The interns and residents at the hospital voted her the best faculty teacher of the year, an honor that helped solidify our role within the academic medical center. I was devastated when Robin returned to MGH, but Tom graciously accepted the full-time position when he completed his residency in the summer of 1988. He devoted the next five years to us, overseeing our 25-bed medical respite program in the Lemuel Shattuck Shelter and our daily clinic at St. Francis House as well as our burgeoning HIV/AIDS services at Boston City Hospital.

Tom was diagnosed with AIDS in 1991, and he taught us all to see this infection through the eyes of our patients. When Tom's energy began to decline a year later, he accepted a position at the Fenway Community Health Center, one of our country's leaders in community-based HIV services.

At dinner we reminisced about our days working together, laughing over stories of our fascinating patients and of the battles we had with so many bureaucracies. Tom reminded me about the 52-year-old man with advanced heart failure who had died unexpectedly in his sleep at the shelter. The shelter staff was so traumatized that a new rule was proposed to not allow anyone over the age of 50 into the shelter. Tom had participated in long meetings and had successfully calmed people by noting that this man would have died on the streets had the shelter not embraced him. He recalled how we would give our patients small alarm clocks in order to take AZT every four hours around the clock. But in our large dormitory-style shelters with so little privacy, these alarms would awaken many folks and identify those with AIDS. Tom's effervescence dissipated as he described the toll that so many premature deaths of our patients had taken on him.

Tom and Rusty both died of complications of AIDS within a month of our dinner. The life-saving highly active anti-retroviral therapy was approved several weeks afterwards in early 1996. The Dr. Tom Bennett Award, our program's highest honor, is given each year to the staff member who embodies Tom's joy and his care and devotion to our poorest neighbors.

Caring for AIDS and other illnesses borne by homeless persons was challenging. Learning to listen to the community after isolated training in an ivory tower was formidable, humbling, and rewarding. The vocal coalition of "stakeholders" that met in 1984-85 to forge a plan for homeless health care services in Boston was comprised of city and state leaders, homeless-service providers and advocates, homeless persons, and representatives from hospitals, neighborhood health centers, and local medical, nursing, and social work schools. Kip Tiernan was the stern but loving taskmaster who became a cherished mentor of mine throughout the formative years of our program. She was the founder of Rosie's Place, the oldest women's shelter in the country, and for many years she was a member of our advisory board. Kip, with characteristic fedora and husky voice and a cigarette lingering from her lower lip, demanded that our program embrace social justice and not charity:

"Never forget that charity is scraps from the table and justice is a seat at the table. First, involve homeless people in all aspects of the program, especially governance. And second, find doctors and nurses who will stay the course and not abandon us after a year or two of doing good work."

A story from 1996 illuminates the convergence of these two edicts. Ellen Dailey, a stately and imposing six-foot-tall African American woman with a booming voice and acerbic wit, was a guest at Long Island Shelter who had several unexplained episodes of passing out, called syncope. Specialists in neurology and cardiology at Boston Medical Center were baffled when all of her blood tests and imaging studies were normal, leaving Ellen discouraged and depressed. Stefan Kertesz, a Harvard Medical School graduate who trained in internal medicine at Beth Israel Hospital in Boston, was one of the doctors in our busy clinic at Long Island Shelter. An astute and attentive clinician, Stefan observed in the shelter something that had not been evident to the specialists—whenever Ellen raised her arms, her heart rate dropped into the low 50s, and she would feel faint. On exam he found that Ellen had a goiter, a thickened and enlarged thyroid. He remembered learning in medical school that a goiter can compress the carotid baroreceptors, causing a precipitous drop in heart rate. Stefan called an endocrinologist at the hospital and explained the urgency of the issue. Ellen was seen soon after and had surgery to remove her thyroid. Ellen's symptoms resolved, and she became Stefan's devoted patient for many years, until he left us to care for homeless persons and to pursue a research career at the University of Alabama, Birmingham. He is now an associate professor of medicine there and is among the most prominent researchers on homeless health care in the nation.

Ellen became the charismatic chair of our consumer advisory board. This board, comprised of homeless persons using our health care services, represents those we serve and meets once each month. Several members of the consumer advisory board are chosen to be part of BHCHP's board of directors, fulfilling our community stakeholders' mandate that homeless persons be directly involved in the governance of our program. With great pride, I would introduce Ellen at local and national meetings as my boss, the person who literally hires and fires us. Ellen attended the annual Health Care for the Homeless Program meetings and helped create a National Consumer Advisory Board that remains dynamic and indispensable. Her experience as a patient in our respite program, including many admissions while she was the vice chair of our board of directors, led her to be a staunch advocate and a founding member of the National Respite Care Providers' Network. Today over 60 cities have respite programs. Ellen was one of two patients each year to share experiences at the white-coat ceremony at Harvard Medical School, exhorting the new medical students to listen to their patients with kindness.

Ellen died suddenly in 2005, and I hope that these stories honor her memory and underscore the sincere appreciation we have for the dedicated homeless persons who continue to inspire and to lead us while serving on our consumer advisory board and our board of directors. Like Kip Tiernan and Barbara McInnis, Ellen Dailey was not satisfied unless we offered homeless persons the very best in health care. Ellen repeatedly bragged that her primary care team in the shelter made a diagnosis that was missed by two prominent specialists. She held all of us to the highest standards, and she insisted that BHCHP be a cradle of excellence and a place where doctors, nurse practitioners, physician assistants, social workers, nurses, and other health professionals could pursue vibrant and rewarding careers.

Poverty's Prism

FEBRUARY 2015

On the evening of October 8, 2014,
I departed Boston on an Aer Lingus
flight to Dublin for an international
street medicine conference and looked
down over Boston Harbor to watch the
buses leave Long Island for the last
time. Mayor Marty Walsh had closed
the crumbling Long Island Bridge
earlier that afternoon and ordered
the entire island evacuated within
four hours. Sisyphus' mythic boulder
rolled down our mountain with a
vengeance that evening.

Built in the 1950s, the bridge had provided the only access to this
harbor island that housed the city's 450-bed emergency shelter and
that was also home to fourteen recovery programs for another 350-
400 homeless persons. I distinctly remember my first ten-mile trek
to the Long Island Shelter clinic in July of 1985: following the path
of the buses from the intake site at Boston City Hospital; crawling
down the choked Southeast Expressway; exiting at Neponset Circle;
hurrying along Quincy Shore Drive past Marina Bay through Squan-
tum to the gate at the guard house; crossing the causeway to Moon
Island; almost veering off the road at the sudden deafening volley of
gunshots coming from the Boston Police Department's firing range
hidden behind a berm; and finally driving across the half-mile bridge.
Unsurprisingly, traffic was restricted to one lane that first night, as
the concrete and steel structure was under repair.

I could not fathom why the city would place a shelter on such an
isolated island, and I conjured images of Father Damien and the leper
colony of Molokai. Such banishment seemed a cruel way to keep this
excluded population out of sight. But like so many others, I was soon
to fall under the island's unique spell.

I made the same journey two evenings a week for the next decade,
during which I worked with a remarkable team of nurses and nurse
practitioners in the bustling shelter clinic that for many individuals
was the first contact with the health care system. Long Island Hospital, a complex of several stunning brick buildings, was opened in 1873
by Boston's Department of Health and Hospitals as the country's first
chronic-care hospital. By the summer of 1985, most of the buildings
were deserted, and the hospital's few remaining patients were housed
in the "runs," three adjacent narrow buildings, each a 26-bed open
ward comprised of thirteen beds along the two long walls with a nurses' station at the entrance and a solarium on the far end. Another early and humbling failure gave me firsthand experience of these "runs."
Ken Taylor, a decorated pilot in the Korean War who had been shot
down and who had spent eight months in a prisoner-of-war camp,
had been sleeping behind the hedges of Old South Church near Co-

pley Square. The worried sexton called on a sweltering August afternoon to ask us to evaluate Ken. Frostbite had claimed part of his foot
the previous winter, and the stump was now weeping malodorous
fluid and crawling with maggots in the summer heat. Flummoxed by
our concern, he begrudgingly agreed to go with us to the emergency
room at Boston City Hospital, where we applied ether to remove the
colony of maggots and placed clean dressings on the stump. Ken then
refused to let us admit him to the hospital for intravenous antibiotics,
and he returned to the streets. Several days later I was called to see
him in the ICU at BCH, where he was intubated and critically ill. The
infection, unchecked by the maggots that kept the wound clean by
eating dead and necrotic skin, had spread to the bloodstream and
caused a collapse of multiple organs. The leg had to be amputated below the knee. He recovered remarkably well, and he was sent to Long
Island Hospital for recuperation. I would visit him each week in the
solarium of his "run," and I listened over chess games to stories of the
horrors suffered by American prisoners in the often forgotten Korean
conflict. I was struck by the lack of privacy in a 26-bed ward, but Ken
taught me the healing value of community and companionship. Ken
never felt alone in the large open room surrounded by hard-working
nurses, aides, and doctors whom he could see and speak to any time
of the day or night. Private and semi-private rooms in our hospitals
can isolate patients, leaving them to wonder when the doctors or
nurses will visit.

In 1983, in response to the growing numbers of homeless persons
in Boston, the Tobin Building, a part of Long Island Hospital that
had once served as Boston's tuberculosis sanatorium and was later
used by the public inebriate program, was converted by Mayor Ray
Flynn to become the city's main shelter. Later I came to understand
that no neighborhood in Boston was willing to support such a large
shelter. The Mayor wisely chose this city-owned island to avoid
NIMBY ("not-in-my-backyard") issues. In addition to withstanding
criticism about exiling homeless people, the Mayor also faced the lo-
gistical nightmare of transporting 450 people in multiple buses each

afternoon from Boston City Hospital and returning them to the city early in the morning.

Long Island is ruggedly beautiful with a panoramic vista across the harbor to the skyline of Boston. Many chose this shelter as respite from the noise and bustle of the city and were willing to queue early to assure a seat on the bus. Two shelter guests living with AIDS showed me the overgrown cemetery with the unmarked graves of hundreds of paupers and indigent Bostonians who had lived in the almshouse that opened in 1882 in a converted hotel on the island. A septuagenarian woman in the shelter foraged for food each evening and fed the growing families of skunks living under the shelter. (The staff soon taught me to dodge these brazen skunks by jiggling my keys as I descended the hill from the parking lot to the shelter.) A man in his early eighties trimmed locks of gray hair from his head each night and sprinkled them into his soup in order "to get enough protein in my diet."

A 1960's modern chapel with vibrantly, if not garishly, colored stained glass overlooked the harbor across from a replica of the grotto of Our Lady of Lourdes in France. The classic lighthouse at the northwest end of the island guided ships into the harbor from the early 1800s—it is still used by pilots approaching Logan airport. A modest two-story house stood a few hundred yards from the shelter in a cluster of pine trees and was rumored to be the "safe house" for sequestering witnesses in the highly publicized federal trial of reputed Mafia crime boss Gennaro Angiulo. At the highest point on the island, just across from the fire station, stands a massive red and white checkered water tower that is visible from downtown Boston. It has rusted in the salt air and been repainted twice in the 30 years since my first visit.

Perhaps my fondest memory of the island was an afternoon in 1988 which we spent hosting Robin Williams and Billy Crystal on a raucous tour of the shelter. The guests were awed and were soon doubled over in peals of laughter as Robin and Billy lambasted them mercilessly with rapid-fire zingers, as only they could do. The lightness and joy of that afternoon was the special gift of these two extraordinary individuals. Together with Whoopi Goldberg and Bob Zmuda, they created Comic Relief with HBO and donated all proceeds to the nineteen health care for the homeless programs originally funded by the Robert Wood Johnson Foundation.

The story of two Long Island Shelter guests in particular has helped me close the chapter on Long Island. Corey Endicott came into the shelter clinic for the first time in September 1985. He was near tears after enduring a barrage of insults for wearing lipstick and painting his fingernails and toenails a deep shade of scarlet. We talked, over several cups of coffee, and he shared how different he always felt from his classmates. At puberty he realized he was gay. He dropped out of high school to escape the daily ridicule, went to Provincetown, and lived with a series of older partners who protected and supported him. This past winter his lover died of AIDS. At the age of 23, Corey was homeless for the first time and found his way to Long Island Shelter. He asked for an HIV test, which was negative. I began to see him regularly to care for his hypertension and migraine headaches.

One evening he proudly introduced me to his new friend Bill Orman, a 37-year-old Vietnam veteran and former Green Beret with a strikingly erect posture and piercing, powder-blue eyes. A weakened muscle caused the right eye to wander to the side, making eye contact uncomfortable. Bill wore combat fatigues and black lace boots and began and ended all responses to me with "sir." A more odd couple I had not seen in the shelter.

Corey and Bill declared proudly one night that they planned to "get married" and have a wedding at the shelter, a gutsy move that won my respect in those contentious years before gay marriages were legalized in Massachusetts in 2004. Politics and religion are passionate topics in the shelters, and I worried about how the other shelter guests would react. The ceremony was held on a beautiful autumn Saturday on the shelter's lawn overlooking the harbor. I had an old camera, and I still cherish the wedding picture of the beaming couple. An unexpected surprise was the nonchalant acceptance and willing participation of many shelter guests in the celebration.

A year later, Corey tested positive for HIV. In those days before highly active anti-retroviral treatment, virtually all of our homeless AIDS patients died of this horrible infection within months. Surprisingly, Corey's immune system remained robust and held the virus in check, placing him in a rare group of people known as long-term non-progressors. Over the ensuing years, Corey vehemently attributed his continued health to a vegetarian diet, including a daily clove of garlic and generous portions of organic greens.

Bill's HIV test remained negative, although he suffered through multiple medical and surgical problems: numbness in both hands required surgery to release the trapped ulna nerves near his elbows; neck and shoulder pain required neurosurgery to stabilize several cervical vertebrae with bulging discs; a small discolored mole on his back proved to be invasive melanoma that required extensive surgery. Bill remained resilient throughout multiple hospital and nursing-home admissions and many prolonged stays in our medical respite facility.

He presented to clinic at Boston City Hospital in 1994 wearing a furry black fedora and black clerical garb, including a Roman collar. He carried a small leather breviary and proudly produced his "ordination" papers, mailed to him after completing a correspondence course that he discovered on the inside flap of a pack of matches.

"I am proud to be Reverend Orman at long last. I have always been an avid Harley Davidson mechanic and I heard my calling to minister to the Hell's Angels, as they deserve a chance to hear about God from one of their own. I spend my days in Revere now, mingling with my old motorcycle friends and preaching the Gospel."

In the early 2000s, Reverend Orman defrocked himself after repeated scuffles with some "church types" on Long Island. He announced that he was now selling commercial real estate in South Boston.

Corey remained healthy and asked often about hormone therapy and the possibility of sexual reassignment surgery. We referred him to the local specialty clinic, and he was bitterly disappointed to be turned down.

"Those assholes think I'm mentally unstable and can't handle all this. I don't care what they think, I am a woman and nothing will change that."

He was distressed about his premature baldness and allowed his fine but sparse strings of remaining hair to grow untamed. He moaned that poverty kept him from the "necessities" of plastic surgery that were so readily available to others.

Corey and Bill stuck together through the years, often coming to clinic together as a couple, bantering and bickering but devotedly holding hands. Bill served as caretaker, constantly worried that Corey was losing weight, isolating himself, or coughing incessantly. Corey relished the attention.

In 2005, they received a "housing first" subsidy and were placed in a sun-filled two-bedroom apartment in Revere. We began to do regular home visits, as we do for all of our chronic rough sleepers who are placed in housing. The apartment was impeccably clean, cluttered with knick-knacks and small mementos, and oppressive with cigarette smoke. They proudly made us tea at each visit and delighted in telling us about their days walking Revere Beach after years in the shelters and on the streets. The wedding photo was on a side table in the living room. One of our great joys has been these "house calls" by our Street Team. We have worked with our housing partners, especially Pine Street Inn and HomeStart, to provide integrated medical- and behavioral-health services directly in the homes of more than 300 of our long-term rough sleepers who have been placed in apartments scattered throughout metropolitan Boston. Our experience with these home visits over the past twelve years has been exhilarating, exhausting, and exasperating. Health and mortality outcomes have been decidedly mixed, while the numbers of street individuals in Boston, as well as in most other major metropolitan cities in the Northeast, have not yet declined as much as we had all so fervently hoped.

Bill called late one night several years ago. He was very concerned and asked us to stop by. Corey had developed fevers, had a hacking cough, and was soaking the sheets with sweat each night. We admitted him to Massachusetts General Hospital with a severe bilateral pneumonia. A blood test showed that his CD4 cell count had plummeted while his HIV viral load had increased dramatically. After twenty years, the virus was now destroying his immune system. Corey improved and was able to go home from the hospital. Despite the trusting relationship we had after so many years, he resisted my ardent and perhaps too strident pleas to begin the medication cocktail that could preserve his life.

"Please don't worry, Doc, I just need to change my diet a little, add a few vitamins and minerals, and I will lick this damn virus."

A week later, Corey was rushed to MGH with *Pneumocystis carini* pneumonia, an AIDS-related opportunistic infection, and he died three days later in the ICU. Bill never left his side and was inconsolable. Over the next several months, we visited Bill often at home. Jim Bonnar, our team's savvy and seasoned psychiatrist, joined us in those visits to help Bill cope with the devastating grief. Bill stopped eating, lost considerable weight, and complained that his whole body was in constant pain. He whispered to me that he didn't see a need to live any longer. He reluctantly agreed to let us admit him to MGH, where we discovered a massive lung cancer that had spread to his bones and his brain. He told us not to worry—he was not afraid and was very anxious to join Corey. Bill Orman, Vietnam veteran, dogged Green Beret, erstwhile minister to Hell's Angels, who dared to marry his lover in a homeless shelter, died peacefully and without pain a week later. In my life as a doctor I have rarely seen such breathtaking love and devotion. Sparked at Long Island Shelter and forged in the crucible of homelessness and abject poverty, the relationship between Bill and Corey survived almost 27 years. Bill and Corey taught me about the pain and suffering of those who have been excluded and cast to the fringes of our society. Both came from hardscrabble poverty, suffered unimaginable physical and sexual abuse as children, and nurtured dreams dashed as their lives spiraled into homelessness. Bill served his country with distinction only to be forgotten on the streets when he came home from Vietnam. In Corey he found a kindred soul too gentle to survive alone on the streets.

Their story spans almost the full arc of my career as a doctor and embodies the joys and frustrations of these past three decades. I was privileged to be invited into their lives and to care for them in the shelters, on the streets, in our respite program, in their homes, and whenever they were hospitalized. Such continuity is a singular gift, a cherished hallmark of BHCHP's philosophy of care, and a major reason we all do this work. Yet the failures linger bitterly, and I remain dismayed that we were unable to convince Corey to take the life-preserving AIDS medications and that we somehow did not discover Bill's cancer until it was untreatable.

A dueling sense of fulfillment and failure has been inescapable. With the help of many partners, we have made remarkable strides in improving the quality, accessibility, and integration of medical and psychiatric care of homeless persons. We have learned to go to people in the shelters and on the streets, to ease their suffering, but never to judge, as we strive for excellence in the care we deliver. Yet we are constantly reminded that the best of health care cannot overcome the powerful social determinants of health.

This winter of 2015 has been particularly frustrating, and we are called to renew our efforts once again. Since the precipitous closing of Long Island, the lack of sufficient shelter and recovery beds and the growing number of people living on the streets are reminiscent of that first winter of 1985. Our fervent hope that Boston's remarkable safety net of emergency shelters and services could be minimized has been temporarily dashed because the stock of available affordable housing has been insufficient to significantly reduce the numbers of chronic shelter and street folks.

I worry that the streets of Boston have grown meaner as our city wearies of a seemingly intractable societal problem. In particular, life for rough sleepers has become more complicated since the closure of the Boston Night Center several years ago. Along with Pine Street Inn's outreach van, the "Nightmare Center," as it was affectionately known, had been the city's lifeline for rough sleepers and the foundation of our street-medicine team since the 1980s. The doors opened at 8:30PM and closed at 5:30AM. No beds or cots were allowed, as the center is not licensed as a "shelter," and as many as 80 men and women were allowed to sleep in chairs or on the floor. A hot meal was served at 9PM, showers and TV were available. Rules were minimal: no weapons, no fighting, no drinking or using drugs on the premises. Violators are asked to leave for an hour, a surprisingly effective behavior-management tool. Street folks were allowed to enter and leave throughout the night, something prohibited in the shelters. Boston's shelters do not allow men and women to be together during the night, one of the reasons that the street population has large numbers of couples. The Boston Night Center permitted men and women to be together, making it a popular life-saving service during the extremes of weather. Shifting state and federal priorities jeopardized funding, and the Boston Night Center closed in 2010 amid optimistic hopes that these rough sleepers would soon be placed in low-threshold supportive housing. Since that time, the plight of street folks has been compounded by restrictions in once friendly public spaces, including Boston Common, Logan Airport, MBTA stations, and our train and bus depots. One hopeful step has been the temporary re-opening of the Boston Night Center by a collaboration of our program with Bay Cove Human Services and Pine Street Inn. As many as 90 persons have sought refuge from the cold and snow each night.

The closure of the Long Island Bridge and the loss of the Boston Night Center offer a poignant glimpse into our past and our future. The island has been set adrift from the mainland by the crumbling of a once sturdy concrete and steel bridge. Seismic upheavals in attitudes have displaced rough sleepers and cast them yet further to the fringes of Boston's urban landscape. After all these years, I accept homelessness as a vexing and complex tragedy that is best seen as a prism held up to our society. Refracted in vivid colors are the weaknesses in each sector, especially housing, education, welfare, labor, health, and justice. Homelessness will never truly be abolished until our society addresses persistent poverty as the most powerful social determinant of health. In the meantime, we must put shoulder to the rock and work together ever more passionately to ease suffering and to seek an end to the injustice of homelessness.

Each day, I pass the framed picture of Corey and Bill on the wall outside my office and see their smiles, although Bill's wandering right eye glances eerily past the camera into some cosmic distance.

Epilogue

In the beginning, I naively planned to devote a year to working with homeless persons and then pursue a career in clinical oncology. Viable career paths in caring for disenfranchised populations were vanishingly rare in academic teaching hospitals. As I slowly came to understand the importance of continuity, consistency, and presence in the care of homeless persons, my dreams of oncology dissipated.

We sought to forge dynamic and sustainable careers for young health professionals seeking to blend clinical work with teaching, education, and research.

BHCHP's work in the shelters and on the streets is fully integrated within the academic teaching hospitals that provide so much acute care to homeless persons. Our doctors share in the care of those admitted to Boston Medical Center and Massachusetts General Hospital, attend on the inpatient medical services of both hospitals, participate in the teaching and training of medical students and residents, and seek ways to be involved in research endeavors that help improve the quality of care of homeless persons. Many of our clinicians have been with us for a decade or longer. Virtually all participated in clinical rotations with us as students and residents, giving us a chance to share our daily work during formative times in their training.

I have worked with hundreds of dedicated people throughout the past 30 years, and space does not allow me to acknowledge them all by name. Our partners at the city, state, and federal level, in the hospitals and academic community, as well as John Lozier and the National Health Care for the Homeless Council, Jim Hunt and the Massachusetts League of Community Health Centers, and everyone throughout the Boston community of shelters, soup kitchens, and homeless services, have blessed us and nurtured us and we could not be more grateful. And no words can capture the gratitude and admiration I have for all of those who have given so much at BHCHP, from clinical to finance to development to human resources to information technology to building services to security to our spectacular kitchen staff. I have a renewed appreciation for the heroic steadfastness of so many of our clinical staff, who go on with remarkable resilience despite the dissolution of so much once taken for granted in our society. They have come to recognize that the lives of those we care for remain vivid, confusing, exasperating, complicated, exhilarating, forgotten, and excluded from the promise of the American dream. That lesson is renewed with each clinical encounter, and BHCHP is blessed with extraordinary staff who persist and even thrive in such difficult and senseless times.

I continue to work as a doctor on our street team, and I would be remiss not to celebrate this special cadre whose dedication to excellence in the care of Boston's chronic rough sleepers brings sheer joy to each day. David Munson completed his residency in medicine at MGH three years ago and inspires me each day with his compassion while teaching me how medicine has evolved over the decades since my own training. Suzanne Armstrong, our extraordinary nurse practitioner and true stalwart of our team, is loved by all on the streets for her humor, kindness, and devotion. Carlos Morales, our newest member, is a gentle and intrepid case worker who keeps us sane with his wizardry in navigating the bureaucratic maze of social service agencies and health plans faced by homeless persons and their caregivers. Jim Bonnar, our beloved psychiatrist and graduate of Harvard College and Harvard Medical School, has taught us to care for those who have suffered unspeakable trauma. Our other psychiatrist is Eileen Reilly, a co-founder of the Women's Lunch Place in the 1980s before finding her way to medical school. After an internship with Dr. Philip Brickner at St. Vincent's Hospital in New York City and residency at the University of Massachusetts in Worcester, Eileen has been a pioneer in taking psychiatry directly to the shelters and streets.

We have been abundantly blessed by the generosity of steadfast donors who have so quietly built and sustained a foundation that has allowed us to dream boldly and to risk failure. We all share the same mission, and all have contributed to what we are today.

Finally, to those who have so graciously invited us into their lives and allowed us to serve them throughout these years, I salute you. I have tried fervently to honor you on every page of this little book.

About the Boston Health Care for the Homeless Program

In 1985, Boston and eighteen other cities across the country were awarded four-year grants through the Health Care for the Homeless Program of the Robert Wood Johnson Foundation and the Pew Charitable Trusts. Modeled upon an innovative program at St. Vincent's Hospital in New York City, these projects were envisioned to be catalysts within the mainstream health care system to improve the accessibility and quality of care provided to homeless persons. The success of this demonstration resulted in the creation of the national Health Care for the Homeless Program of the Bureau of Primary Health Care, Health Resources and Services Administration, US Department of Health and Human Services. Over 240 projects in cities within every state as well as Puerto Rico and the Virgin Islands are currently funded under this program.

BHCHP embraces a mission of assuring access to the highest quality health care for homeless persons in the greater Boston area. The foundation of the service-delivery model has been interdisciplinary teams of physicians, nurse practitioners, physician assistants, nurses, social workers, and community support workers who conduct daily clinics at two major teaching hospitals, Boston Medical Center and Massachusetts General Hospital. These teams then offer direct health care services at over 65 sites, including adult and family shelters, shelters for victims of domestic abuse, soup kitchens and day centers, detoxification units and corrections facilities, the backstretch barns of a local thoroughbred racetrack, directly on the streets, and even "house calls" to several hundred formerly homeless persons who have been placed in supportive housing.

BHCHP's innovative medical respite program, the 104-bed Barbara McInnis House, offers acute, sub-acute, pre- and post-operative, recuperative, palliative, and end-of-life care to individuals too ill or infirm to withstand the rigors of survival on the streets and in the shelters.

Homeless persons are fully involved in strategic planning and governance, as members of BHCHP's Board of Directors and an active Consumer Advisory Board. BHCHP provides integrated medical, oral, mental health, and addictions care for more than 12,000 homeless men, women, and children each year.

About the Author

A native of Newport, Rhode Island, Jim O'Connell graduated from the University of Notre Dame in 1970 and received a master's degree in theology from Cambridge University in 1972. After earning an M.D. from Harvard Medical School in 1982, he completed a residency in Internal Medicine at Massachusetts General Hospital. O'Connell began full-time clinical work with homeless individuals as a founding physician of the Boston Health Care for the Homeless Program in 1985.

Under his leadership, BHCHP has grown to be a vital and dynamic presence in the continuum of care for poor and marginalized populations in Boston and has pioneered many innovations, including the nation's first medical respite program in 1985, the transition to funding as a federally qualified health center in 1988, and implementation of the first electronic medical record for a health care for the homeless program in collaboration with the Laboratory of Computer Science of MGH in 1996. Dr. O'Connell shares a particular passion for the care of "rough sleepers," and street medicine has been integral to BHCHP's model of care since 1985. He currently juggles a busy clinical role on the program's street team with his duties as President of BHCHP.

The recipient of many prizes and awards, including the Albert Schweitzer Humanitarian Award in 2012 and The Trustees' Medal at the bicentennial celebration of MGH in 2011, Dr. O'Connell is Assistant Professor of Medicine at Harvard Medical School. He has lectured internationally, and his research has been published in a broad array of journals. He lives with his family in Dorchester, Massachusetts. This is his first book.

Acknowledgements

Stories from the Shadows would not have been possible without the steadfast encouragement of two cherished colleagues, Bob Taube and Barry Bock, and our Board of Directors: Larry Adams, Sarah Anderson, Bruce Bullen, Barbara Blakeney, Tom Dehner, Joanne Guarino, Dr. Chris Latham, Steve Lipiner, Kevin Leary, Brett Painchaud, Hap Redgate, Dr. Lisa Rubinstein, Len Simons, Dr. Brian Swann, Steve Tringale, and Derek Winbush.

I especially want to celebrate the lives of four persons who devotedly served BHCHP: John Griffin, Louise Mercurio, and Michael Reynolds, consumers of our services and energetic members of our Board of Directors, and Jay Tankanow of our Consumer Advisory Board. We have been left bereft by their deaths over these past two years and this book honors their memory.

This has been a labor of love that would not have been possible without the devotion, muse, forbearance, and determination of four extraordinary mid-wives. Linda O'Connor has been a resolute and ever-so-gentle source of encouragement, Mala Rafik our legal and wise counsel, Margaret Boles Fitzgerald the irrepressible force of gravity that has kept this project grounded, and Sarah Anderson my *alter ego* who has walked each step of this journey and always been there for me. My sincere and heartfelt thanks to all of you.

Years of cherished monthly dinners with my close friend Mark L. Wolf, Senior Judge and former Chief Judge of the United States District Court, District of Massachusetts nourished this book. An astute master of law and poetry, devoted to family, and passionate about service to the poor and disenfranchised, Mark's probing insight and steadfast encouragement kept this dream alive. I could not be more grateful.